THE ART OF EATING
WITHOUT A STOMACH

HOW TO THRIVE AFTER GASTRECTOMY
FOR STOMACH CANCER

DR. PETER THATCHER

The Art of Eating Without a Stomach

© 2014 Dr. Peter Thatcher,
All rights reserved.

TABLE OF CONTENTS

INTRODUCTION

Your New Life After Gastrectomy

Gastrectomy.

You have been through one of the worst experiences a person can ever have to endure. To have your stomach removed was a massive undertaking. But you've come out the other side, not only alive, but with a greater verve for life and really living than you ever thought was possible. Stomach cancer decided to do battle with you, and even though it may have ravaged your body and changed your life, you are *alive*.

Despite needing to go through a gastrectomy and losing a portion, or all, of your stomach, you were able to beat it.

That was the tough part, but *you did it*.

Now, you need to adjust to the changes in your life when it comes to your diet. There will be changes, no doubt about it. You have likely lost a substantial amount of weight as well. However, if you've made it this far, you can do anything, and that includes changing the way you eat and the types of food you eat.

Fortunately, the changes are not so "over the top" that you won't be able to handle them. You don't have to go on a liquid diet, and you don't have to subsist solely on supplements and intravenous fluids.

You can still eat. You can still enjoy food and make a variety of different recipes that have been a staple of your diet for years. While you must cut out a few things, such as all of those sweets, you should still be able to enjoy many of your favorites.

Through the course of this book, I will illustrate the foods you should and should not eat and the complications you might encounter; how often and how much you should eat; and I will even toss in some tasty and simple recipes for you to add to your collection.

Even though you will be changing your diet and your lifestyle, it doesn't mean you have to stop enjoying life or stop enjoying food. You survived, and now it's time to get on with really living. This book aims at helping you to do just that.

CHAPTER 1

Gastrectomy Changes Your Life and the Way You Eat

As a stomach cancer patient who has undergone a gastrectomy, you will find that the procedure will change your life, In particular, it will change the way you have to eat. Throughout this book, I will examine your post op dietary life in every aspect, from the reasons it is important to start eating again, to the foods you should eat and avoid. The advice and tips in the book, along with some tasty recipes, should help you to learn that even though going through a gastrectomy will change your life, it will not ruin your life.

Follow Some Simple Rules for Life after Gastrectomy

After you have undergone a full or partial gastrectomy and you begin to heal, it can be quite challenging to follow a good and proper new dietary regimen.

Post-surgery, it is extremely important for you to be as careful as possible of the postoperative area, and it is important to start eating as soon as you are able.

This can be difficult for some, but the following tips and simple rules should help you on your way. Those who go through the surgery tend to lose a substantial amount of bodyweight – around 20%, or more in some cases. It is vital to remedy this drastic weight loss, but it is also important to make sure you do this the *right* way. You must ensure you are getting enough nutrients from the foods you are eating so you do not continue to lose weight.

Eat Smaller Meals More Frequently

Instead of trying to eat three large main meals, which will simply not be possible as you no longer have a stomach to hold your food, it makes far more sense to eat five to six smaller meals throughout the day. By eating every couple of hours and by keeping the meals very small, you will retrain your body to digest properly.

Even though you are eating smaller meals, you will be eating more times throughout the day, so you will still be able to get enough nutrients into your body.

Chew Well and Eat Slowly

As you begin this new chapter in your dietary history, always make sure you are chewing your food completely. More chewing breaks the food down further, and thus will make it easier for your body to digest.

It is also a good idea to eat slowly. When you eat slowly, your brain and body work better together to let you know when you are full. This ensures you do not eat more than you should in one sitting. You don't want to eat too much at once because it can cause discomfort and even pain, which can make you want to eat less and less, thus resulting in more unwanted weight loss.

Drinking

When it comes to drinking with your meals, you have two options. Choose the one that works the best for you:

1. Wait to have a drink between thirty and sixty minutes after eating solid food—for some this is the best option for avoiding nausea and potential irritation of the postoperative area.
2. Drink with your meals, but limit your liquid intake at this time to around four ounces. This ensures you will still get enough solid food without the liquid making you feel full

before you really are.

My best advice is to try both methods to see which one works the best for you. Of course, ultimately, you will want to heed the advice of your own doctor, dietician or nutritionist, too.

Keep a Food Diary

Start keeping a food diary so you can track what foods you are eating and in what amount. Then record how you feel. This will allow you to see what foods you can eat and which foods your body now finds intolerable, as everyone is a bit different. It also lets you calculate whether you are actually getting enough nutrients throughout the day.

You may also find it advantageous to get in touch with a dietician or nutritionist who has experience with gastrectomy patients.

Working with someone who specializes in creating diets specific to your condition is not always necessary, as you will be able to put together an excellent dietary plan on your own once you have finished reading this book. However, some find it beneficial to have the guidance of a professional to help them along the way.

Support and Encouragement from Family and Friends

You are going through some rather large changes in your life, and it is important to have a great support team there who can help you make it through all of those changes as happy and healthy as possible.

Your family and friends are essential in this. In Chapter 10, I will be discussing how to deal with various social situations after a gastrectomy, as well as how you can speak with your family about your new dietary plan and needs.

Once you have a great team on your side, you'll find that sticking to the plan and gaining back that weight is possible, and it might even be easier than you thought it would be!

Summary

After you go through a gastrectomy, your life will change and your eating habits will be forever altered. Despite the changes, it does not mean the end of your life, the end of enjoying the taste of food, or the end of your social outings with family and friends.

You still have *plenty* of options.

Follow the simple tips in this book, and you will learn to eat healthy and eat right after your gastrectomy.

CHAPTER 2

The Importance of Eating and Regaining Your Weight

After a gastrectomy, it can be very difficult for people to maintain the necessary nutritional intake and caloric intake needed to regain bodyweight. As mentioned, this type of procedure will cause drastic weight loss in the vast majority of people who go through the process.

Thus, it becomes important to regain the lost weight and to maintain a good and healthy weight. Some people have a substantial amount of trouble with this thought.

In this chapter, I will show you the importance of eating and the reasons why you need to regain your weight. I will also look at some of the difficulties that many people have when they attempt this and ways that you can alleviate some of those difficulties in your own attempt.

What Does the Stomach Really Do?

To understand the gastrectomy and the role it ultimately plays in your nutrition, it is important to have a good idea of what the stomach really does. It stores food and is important in the digestive process, but only a small amount of the nutrition from food actually absorbs into the body when it is in the stomach.

Most people do not realize this, and they believe that most of the digestion happens in the stomach. The stomach is where enzymes mix with the food that aid in the process of digestion. The majority of the nutrient absorption actually comes when food passes through the intestines.

Without a stomach, or with only a partial stomach, it becomes more difficult to eat and utilize those calories. However, by changing the way that you eat and altering the things that you eat, it does become possible.

By eating the right types of foods, including calorie dense foods, it is possible to enjoy a good and healthy diet that ensures you will not lose any more weight, and that you are able to regain some of that weight that you lost.

Why Gain Weight?

You've gone through cancer and now you are trying to get better and heal, and a part of that needs to be regaining the weight you've lost leading up to and after the gastrectomy.

The entire world seems obsessed with ways to drop weight, and they pay good money to shed the unwanted pounds. These types of problems are ones that cancer sufferers wished they had.

Cancer wreaks havoc on the body, and it can be debilitating and deadly. People who have cancer have different requirements and diets because they need to be able to keep up their strength. Adding even *more* protein and calories to the diet becomes important. It helps you to stay strong, literally.

Issues with Fast Weight Loss

One of the hallmarks of losing weight with a gastrectomy is that the weight loss is rapid, and this can lead to a number of health problems, such as gallstones and even liver damage. Fast weight loss can also change your hormonal balance.

Rapid weight loss can also throw off the fluid balance in your body. Your muscles depend on proper electrolyte balance in the body. This can be difficult to maintain during rapid weight loss and for those who are underweight. This can often be quite damaging to the heart, which is one of the most important muscles of the body.

Gaining weight and keeping it becomes highly important for the overall health of a gastrectomy patient. It ensures you retain proper muscle mass and that you have a healthy body able to handle the stresses you've gone through with cancer and recovery.

People who go through the gastrectomy often have trouble when it comes to getting their body back to what they consider "normal." It does take time for an appetite to return, but with the right attitude, the right process, and some good recipes, it will soon return.

Your Changing Tastes

One of the other things that can cause many people to stop eating is that their tastes change. Sometimes, the foods they once liked simply no longer appeal to them (a curious and largely unexplained phenomena), and the desire to eat goes away.

This happens to many people who have a gastrectomy, and it is normal. Dealing with this issue will take some creativity and some experimentation. While it is possible to force yourself to eat foods that you find no longer taste good just for the caloric value, this diminishes the joy that you should *still* experience from eating your meals.

Continue to go back and try those foods you once loved but don't have a taste for now. Keep in mind that your tastes could change yet again, and you might find that you are once again enjoying those foods.

But it's also time to try some new foods that your taste buds might now enjoy a bit more. Try some new types of foods and find options that you really do enjoy. The recipes in this book should help to give you a good variety of options to try. If you find several foods that you enjoy and that are good for you, they will likely become the staples of your new diet, at least for a time.

Keep experimenting and finding new and interesting foods that will keep you coming back for more.

You Don't Feel Like Eating

One of the other problems that many people who have undergone a gastrectomy face is they don't have an appetite. When they don't feel like eating, they don't bother thinking about their nutritional needs, and they skip meals. This becomes dangerous. Without the proper nutrition and calories, more weight loss will occur, and additional health issues will surely follow.

You must enter into the mindset that even if you do not feel like eating, it is still essential to eat so you can get the nutrients and the calories your body needs. By understanding and adhering to a set schedule, your body will eventually become used to the process of eating and digesting. Again, this process will take time.

While you should not force yourself to eat if you actually feel full and as though you *can't* eat any more, you should always make sure you eat at specific times on your daily schedule.

Setting Up a Daily Schedule

One of the best ways to make sure you adjust to life after a gastrectomy is to set up and stick to a schedule. Having an eating schedule that you can look at and adhere to daily provides you with some accountability, and for many people this makes it easier to eat right and to regain weight.

Tips for Creating Your Plan

I will go into detail about meal plans and recipes later, but it's important to know how to schedule a basic meal plan, and how setting up a meal plan for someone who has had a gastrectomy differs from other meal plans out there.

It is important to remember that those other meal plans do not account for your changing lifestyle and your surgery, so they will *not* be ideal for you.

Your plan must accommodate your specific needs, and that means you will not be eating just three or four meals a day. Instead, you will want to have smaller meals, and you will generally want to have between five and six of these smaller meals throughout the day.

Spreading them out from morning to early evening ensures your body has a full supply of calories and nutrition throughout the day, and that you are still digesting the food properly.

When you create your plan, you will want to have specific times set up at which you should eat. Now, it's important to remember that *each person* is unique when it comes to the times that he or she wants to eat. You have to base the plan on your own schedule.

Some people wake later in the day, so they start their first meal later. Once you have the time for the first meal of the day, you will then want to have your subsequent meals every two hours or so.

Changing Schedules

Sometimes, you may find that your schedule changes. Maybe you are on a trip or you are changing your sleep pattern. Simply adjust the first meal of the day to a new time, and then continue with the eating schedule of every one to two hours thereafter, and your body should not notice a difference.

Make Your Food Work *for* You

Over the course of the rest of the book, I will delve into a variety of recipes and options you have for adding food to your diet that you actually like and that have enough calories to ensure you are putting on and maintaining a healthy weight.

The real key behind this thought is to make sure your foods are working for you. What does this mean? In a nutshell, it means that you have to think about what it is that you are eating.

While those who are intentionally trying to lose weight will drink water as a means to feel full before they start actually eating food, you will want to do the opposite. Instead of drinking water before a meal or with a meal, consider adding a drink that adds actual calories and nutrients. Smoothies, for example, are a good option, and later I will go over a number of great and tasty recipes you can try.

High calorie, nutrient rich foods are always the way to go, since you will be eating smaller portions at a time and eating more throughout the day.

I will cover some of the best types of food to eat on this diet in later chapters in the book.

How Often Should You Get on the Scale?

While it is important to monitor your weight while trying to gain, it's also important not to obsess over the scale. Most of the time, when people are trying to lose weight, they hear that they should not step on the scale too often, as there will be weight fluctuations and it can sometimes become discouraging.

The same is true when it comes to gaining weight. If you spend too much time worrying about the scale rather than focusing on eating healthy, high calorie foods, and find that your progress is not what you hoped, it can derail you.

Weighing yourself *is* important though, as it can let you know what is working and what is not working in your weight gain plan. It lets you know if you are on track to gain back your weight.

I recommend that you get on the scale every week or every couple of weeks and record your progress in your food diary. That way, you can compare your weight gained to what foods you ate during that time. If you find that you are eating often, but you are not gaining weight, then you may need to revisit the types of foods and drinks you are eating.

Also, speak with your doctor, dietician or nutritionist about how often you should weigh yourself. Many will actually be interested to see just how quickly you are able to progress, and they will want to monitor your weight gain while you are healing and trying to get on with normal eating habits after the surgery. It helps them gauge just how well you are doing, and they can help you make changes to your regimen as needed.

When you do weigh yourself, make sure you are doing so at the same time of day. Small fluctuations in the body can cause your weight to differ morning, midday and evening, so keep the times that you weigh yourself the same, just so you have the most accurate possible data.

The Power of Positive Thinking

Cancer and cancer treatment fall firmly into the realm of nature and science. The treatments for cancer and for dealing with life after a gastrectomy tend to fall into the scientific realm, as well. However, positive thinking can play quite an important role as well, even though "good thoughts" and positive thinking are certainly anything but scientific.

It is important to understand how vital positive thinking really can be. Even though your life may have changed, it is important for you to remember that at least you still have a life. Many cancer patients are not as lucky as you.

By remaining as positive as possible, and by focusing on getting healthier, it becomes possible to start to feel much better about your situation. When you genuinely feel better in your mind, your body can feel better as well.

One of the biggest benefits is that it can keep you from dwelling on the negative, and there is likely plenty of negativity swimming through your mind right now. Positive thoughts help to banish that negativity and depression that it brings through.

Though there is no substitute for proper medical treatment and eating right to regain your strength and health, positive thinking can make a real difference in your life, so always try to look for the bright side and try to enjoy your life as much as possible.

However, staying positive is not always an easy thing to do. Here are some quick tips that you should keep in mind to help you keep on the positive side of life as much as you can. They really can help when you are dealing with these types of issues, so don't ignore them.

Tips for Thinking Positive

- Focus on all of the *good* things happening in your life right now.
- Smile.
- Set goals for eating more and gaining back your weight and for other things you want to do with your life.
- Look at each additional day with your family and friends as a gift.
- Express your creativity.
- Live in the moment.
- Listen to uplifting music.
- Read uplifting and positive books.
- Surround yourself with loving and positive people.
- Do not focus on the negatives.

Summary

Gaining weight is essential if you want to return to being as healthy as you possibly can after going through the gastrectomy. The drastic weight loss suffered after a gastrectomy can be devastating on the body, and even dangerous. You lose muscle tissue, and this can affect the strength of your heart. Your liver and other internal organs can take damage as well, so it is essential that you take steps as soon as you can to start regaining that lost weight.

Even though it can be difficult to get onto the right type of plan, and it takes time to regain the weight you've lost, you *can do it*.

By setting up a proper eating schedule, finding types of foods that are good for your new lifestyle and that you enjoy, and by keeping as positive as possible, you can make some real changes that will help you regain that weight.

CHAPTER 3

Foods to Eat and Foods to Avoid

When you've had a gastrectomy, you will find that you can tolerate some types of foods better than you can tolerate other types of food. In this chapter, I will go over the typical foods you will want to be eating and adding to your diet, as well as the foods you should avoid.

Tolerances May Vary

Remember that some people may have different tolerances, and that those tolerances may change over time. Always pay attention to how you are feeling after you eat, and pay attention to any side effects or issues that happen after eating and during digestion.

Later in the book, I will go over some of the health issues that you may face while returning to eating after a gastrectomy, including a condition known as dumping syndrome. By paying attention to these things, as well as how you feel in general after eating, you will be able to develop a list of foods ideal for you.

After you've undergone this procedure, it is true that the foods you eat may be different foods from those you were eating before. However, you will still be able to enjoy many of the same options, and you can always find some delicious recipes to try.

The following are the various types of foods you should and should not be eating after the surgery. Keep these lists in mind when you are shopping, when you are eating out at a restaurant, or when you are over at a friend's house.

In addition to a variance in your tolerances, you may also find that your tastes change, and they can even change from day to day. Understand that this happens with many patients, and you simply need to have an array of different foods on hand that you typically enjoy, and that are good for you.

A Different Type of Diet

One of the things you will notice about these suggested foods is that I don't tell you that you can't eat certain types of foods that other diets might tell you to avoid because of calories, or because they aren't typically "healthy" according to fitness experts who are trying to get their clients to drop weight. *That's not the purpose of this type of dietary lifestyle.*

The foods on this plan are perfectly good for you, and I will show you foods that are full of calories and nutrients. This means that cream and butter are on the menu. You are trying to put on some weight, so you want foods full of calories. However, that does not mean you want to have sweet food in your diet.

People who have had stomach cancer and who have gone through a gastrectomy will want to have a diet a particular ratio:

- Higher in protein.
- Lower in carbohydrates.

You should also avoid sweets. Calories are good; *sweets* are bad. In some cases though, you may need to have a small amount of sugar to help balance your blood sugar levels. Talk with your doctor, dietician or nutritionist about the correct level of sugar you need to have in your diet.

The addition of sauces and gravy to food is a good way to add some extra calories without adding too much to the actual physical portion of the food.

Breads and Grains

You will still be able to enjoy many different types of breads and grains, although you will want to avoid some of the options out there. See my list for specifics.

Foods to Eat
- Whole grain breads
- Bagels
- Crackers
- Unsweetened cereal
- Pasta
- Rice
- Barley
- Potatoes
- Popcorn
- Pretzels

Foods to Avoid
- Sweetened muffins
- Pastries
- Sugary cereals
- Cake
- Doughnuts

Fruits

While you might think that all fruits would naturally be good for you, there are some you will actually want to avoid now that you've undergone this surgery.

Foods to Eat
- Fresh fruit – any of your favorites should do nicely
- Canned fruit – but make sure it is not in heavy syrup and that there is no added sugar
- Frozen fruit – again, you don't want anything with sugar added to it

Foods to Avoid
- Canned fruit in syrup
- Dried fruit
- Sweetened fruit juice
- Pie filling from a can

Vegetables

Most of the time, vegetables are going to be great for you and they will be the smart choice. However, just like the fruits, you will need to avoid some vegetables.

Foods to Eat
- Fresh and frozen – all vegetables that are your favorites

Foods to Avoid
- Vegetables with additional sugars or sweet sauces – mainly, these are things to avoid when preparing the veggies and to ask about when you are going out to eat somewhere

Meat and Protein

One of the great things about meat and protein is that most people who have had a gastrectomy have little trouble when it comes to eating and digesting them. Try a variety of different types of protein to see which ones you enjoy the most.

Even if you are a vegetarian, you should still be able to discover quite a few great options.

Foods to Eat
- Beef
- Lamb
- Venison
- Chicken
- Turkey
- Fish
- Seafood
- Peanut butter
- Dried peas
- Nuts
- Beans
- Cheese
- Eggs
- Milk
- Cottage cheese
- Plain yogurt

Foods to Avoid

None. You are good to go to try any protein for your diet. As with other foods, start out with these proteins slowly just so you can see how everything you put into your body makes you feel after eating.

Fats and Oils

Despite what some might think, you definitely need to have some fats and oils in your diet if you want to remain healthy. This is particularly true when it comes to someone who is trying to maintain or regain weight.

Of course, some types of fats and oils are better for you than others are, so adhere to the following lists.

Foods to Eat

- Butter
- Margarine
- Mayonnaise
- Cream
- Sour cream
- Salad dressing

Foods to Avoid

- Honey butter
- Salad dressings that contain honey
- Sweet cream cheese

Sweets/Desserts

Just because you are on a different dietary regimen, it does not mean you have to forego some of the sweeter things in life. As you've seen from the other items in this list, it does mean you need to be a bit more careful about the things you are putting into your body.

When it comes to sweets and desserts, always look for the sugar free options and substitutes.

Foods to Eat
- Sugar free cake and cookies
- Sugar free ice cream
- Sugarless gum
- Fruit preserves
- Low/no sugar jelly

In general, look for options that say low sugar or sugar free on the labels to be on the safe side.

Foods to Avoid
- Ice cream
- Cake
- Frosting or Icing
- Cookies
- Candy
- Syrup

Just as you want to look for the sugar free options for your diet, you need to avoid those foods that have sugar in them.

While this constitutes many items that fall into the sweets category, there really are plenty of great and tasty sugar free options out there today. These alternate choices will satisfy any sweet cravings you might have while still being a food your system will be able to tolerate.

As much as you may want and feel as though your taste buds crave the actual sugar, avoid it. Look for alternatives, such as a sweet piece of fresh fruit, or even a piece of sugarless gum.

Beverages

With beverages, you have some leeway with what you drink, but again, you will want to stay away from anything sweetened. In the next chapter, I will show you how much you should drink throughout the day, and when you should drink.

Drinks to Choose

- Water
- Coffee
- Tea
- Milk
- Broth
- Soft drinks with artificial sweeteners

Drinks to Avoid

- Sweetened soda
- Sweetened tea and coffee
- Lemonade
- Kool-Aid
- Chocolate milk and traditional sweetened milkshakes
- *Any* sweetened beverages

The Nutrients You Need

The foods that are tolerable for most full and partial gastrectomy patients outlined in the lists above are *full* of nutrients and calories, which should make it possible to eat and maintain a healthy body.

Stomach cancer sufferers will do better when they have extra vitamin D, iron, and calcium in their diets. Many times, you will be able to get the additional nutrients from milk, cheese, cabbage, broccoli, bread, sardines, and other foods. However, your doctor may also recommend taking additional supplements, especially in the early days of getting the body accustomed to eating once again.

In the later chapters, I will cover some tasty recipes that utilize these basic types of foods and that avoid sweet foods so you can have a truly diverse meal plan that never gets boring for you!

It Takes Time

Do all of these "rules" about the foods you should and should not be eating sound confusing? If so, then you are certainly not alone. In the beginning, many people find it difficult to understand just what they should and should not ingest after their gastrectomy.

Using these lists, and taking the time to see how each of the different foods makes you feel after eating it, can make a real difference. It takes a bit of time, but you will be able to discover just what foods are right for you and will help you gain and maintain a healthy weight.

Tips for Eating

The foods outlined here are good options for those who are healing from their surgery and trying to gain weight. However, it is just as important to learn just how to eat properly again while using these foods. Your experiences may vary from those of other sufferers, but the following tips should be helpful in making sure you are on the right path and that you can keep the food down.

Fiber Rich Foods – Pros and Cons

Choosing foods that are high in fiber, such as whole wheat bread and grains, can be a good idea for people. However, they do tend to make some people feel full faster. They can make some people feel uncomfortably full, which means people will stop eating before they get enough calories and nutrients.

It may be a good idea to reduce the amount of high fiber foods, beans, lentils, and leafy greens that can give you the feeling of being full too soon.

Others will find that they have no trouble with these carbohydrates, and that they can eat grains and leafy vegetables without any uncomfortable feelings. For those people, have at those foods and enjoy them!

Bland Food May Be Your Friend

Often, those who have gone through cancer have problems with nausea, and this is certainly true of people who have had a gastrectomy. Dealing with this problem can make regaining weight quite tricky. However, you can do some things to make it a bit easier for you.

Choosing to eat foods typically thought of as bland can be a very good way to combat this nausea.

Another way that some people have had success in dealing with nausea is to eat food at room temperature. This reduces the odor and the taste, two of the main contributing factors to nausea in stomach cancer sufferers.

If you feel that you continually have a "bad" taste in your mouth that lasts between meals, it can make eating that next meal a real chore. A way to combat this problem is to have a sugar free mint that can neutralize the taste.

Sour Might Work for You

Sweet foods should be something you avoid when you are creating your new diet plan. Although sweets might not be on your menu, that doesn't mean you can't enjoy some tart and sour foods.

In fact, they might be a nice addition if you have issues with vomiting. The sour foods such as vinegar, lemon, lime, grapefruit, cranberry, salsa and pickles are often easier for you to keep down, as are the bland foods.

Experiment with Foods

Take your time to experiment with different types of foods and different preparation methods to find out what you like the most. Determine what you find most appealing when it comes to the taste, as well as when it comes to the texture and the smell of the food.

By learning to make the food appetizing to you and your new tastes, rather than simply choosing to make foods the same way you've always made them, they can become appealing again.

This is particularly important for those who have been having trouble suffering from nausea with foods they once loved. A few tweaks here and there to your favorite recipes, and you could be back in business!

Simple Tips to Make Your Food Tastier and Full of Calories

Since you are trying to regain weight, and you want to have some food that tastes great, consider trying these two simple and effective tips to give your food some added flavor as well as some added punch in the calorie department.

Marinate It

A great way to improve the taste of fish, chicken, and meat is with a marinade of your choice, so long as it is not sweet and sugary. You can buy premade marinates or create your own. I'll include a couple of simple sugar free marinade recipes in the later chapters that you can try, too!

This gives you some extra taste, and it gives you a few added calories, which as so important when you are trying to gain back that weight you lost during your treatment and surgery.

Add Some Bacon Bits

If you are having vegetables, some fresh salad, soup, or nearly anything else for that matter, adding bacon bits might be a nice idea. You can make your own bacon bits if you like, or you can use the ones found at the grocery store.

They add some calories from fat and a bit of protein, and they can make even what you would normally consider a bland salad taste fantastic.

Consider Commercial Supplements

Something else you might want to consider is looking into some of the commercial supplements on the market for weight gain. Always make sure you look at the ingredients so you can ascertain whether they are full of sugar or not, naturally.

Many of the supplements on the market today, such as Boost, Carnation Instant Breakfast, Build-up, Complan and some of the various weight gain powders that bodybuilders use could be a *very good* addition to your pantry.

If you are going to choose some of the commercial products out there, it pays to do a bit of research first. In addition to checking the ingredients and making sure sugar isn't a part of it, you will also want to consider the taste.

Some of the protein powders out on the market today taste good, or at least passable. However, other types and brands have a definite "bad" taste, or at least many people consider it bad. You may also not enjoy the texture. It might be gritty, or it might have a foul aftertaste.

Since your taste buds may be more sensitive and you may be pickier after surgery, it might be a good idea to consider looking at some reviews to see what people say about the taste. It's also a good idea to buy a smaller container of the product to try before you go all out and buy a big bucket of the stuff!

If you can handle it, commercial protein powders can be a very good way to get some extra calories and protein relatively easily. And while you're blending up a batch, throw in some fruits and vegetables for added nutrients!

Improve Your Oral Health

While this might sound a bit strange, improving your oral health really can help with your appetite. Many times, when people are suffering from cancer and dealing with the aftermath of a gastrectomy, they fall into something of a depression. This is natural for many people.

Some neglect to take care of some of their other personal health needs because they feel so focused on the cancer. Again, this is a natural response. Suddenly, things such as brushing your teeth each night don't matter when you are dealing with the reality of cancer.

Now that you are getting your body and your health back on track, you will find that better oral health can actually help your appetite. By having a clean mouth, through brushing and flossing, food can taste better.

Make sure you visit the dentist or oral hygienist as well, just to make sure there are no other issues with your oral health. Some people have changed senses of taste and smell after going through cancer treatment and having a gastrectomy, so the dentist can make sure that your loss of taste and smell is not a dental issue.

As Always, Talk With Your Doctor

While these suggestions for foods to eat and foods to avoid are all good options, before you create a diet plan after gastrectomy, you should always consult with your doctor first, just to make sure you are going to be getting enough calories in the plan. They may have their own specialized plan for their patients that you should try.

As mentioned earlier, you can also work with a dietician or nutritionist who has experience helping cancer patients who have no stomach or a partial stomach. They will be able to help monitor your progress, as well.

Summary

The foods that you eat on your new diet are not necessarily going to be vastly different from the foods that you ate before, but as you can see from the items listed in this chapter, you will have to deal with some changes to the way you eat and the foods you cook.

Are these the only foods that you can eat after a gastrectomy? Not at all! However, these are the basics that you will likely want to start with as you learn what your body will and will not tolerate.

You can use the list in this chapter as a guideline when you are heading to the grocery store and shopping.

CHAPTER 4

How Much Should You Eat and How Often

One of the biggest questions and concerns people will have once they come home and start healing from their surgery is just how much they should eat and how often they should have their meals.

After you have surgery, and while you are still in the hospital, you will start on soft foods, such as applesauce, cooked cereal, cottage cheese, bananas, sugar free pudding and plain or sugar free yogurt.

Once you are able to do well with these types of soft foods, your doctor will then suggest that you move on to start eating solid foods again. This process does take some adjusting, as you can imagine, but once you start to eat regular food again, you will be able to start regaining that weight.

How Often Should You Have Your Meals?

As I mentioned earlier, you will not be eating large meals three times a day as you once did. Instead, eating between five and six smaller meals per day is a better option. It ensures you are getting enough calories, and it ensures you are not putting too much pressure on your diminished capacity to ingest food at the time.

At the end of the chapter, I will show you a sample meal plan that will give you a basic idea of how you can split up your meals through the day.

This meal plan is not set in stone, naturally, and you can certainly make small adjustments to accommodate your lifestyle needs.

Find the Time

Ideally, you will be able to have five to six times daily when you can sit down for a small meal or snack. It does not take long to eat and to make sure you have enough calories in your body to sustain you.

If you are still working, you will find that many employers will accommodate you. Just explain your situation and nutrition requirements. If you aren't working and you are at home, then it should be relatively easy to set up a schedule you can stick to with your diet. If you find it hard to stick to it on your own, then find someone who can support you and you can talk to.

Of course, this all depends on your personal situation. No matter what's happening in your life, you need to find the time to take good care of your health. Make sure you find the time to eat throughout the day and *always* try to stick to your eating schedule.

Separating the Meals

Your first meal should generally occur within about an hour or two after waking. Of course, some people tend to feel a bit nauseous upon first waking, and the last thing they are thinking about is eating.

Get up and get ready for the day, and let your body get acclimated a little bit before eating. However, you should not let more than two hours go by after waking before you have your first meal.

One other thing to note is that many nutritionists who are creating typical diet plans for people who are *not* in your situation will have plans that consist of having very large meals as your first meal of the day. Ignore those diet plans that you see all over the web. Your first meal should be small.

You will generally be eating the same or similar sized meals throughout the day to reach your caloric goal. Eating too much in one sitting can be painful, and this could cause you to want to skip meals later, which you simply can't do.

Through the Day

Try to eat every hour and a half to two hours. You may find that you need to add or reduce the time between meals to meet your hunger levels. However, you should never wait too long between meals – no more than two to three hours. If you don't feel hungry, at least try to have a small snack, just so you can make sure you are getting the calories you need. Always have snacks on hand, whether you are staying home or going out.

A good way to make sure you are getting those additional calories, even when you aren't eating a normal meal, is by having a smoothie. Having one of these for a meal, and as a snack "between" meals, will provide you with more calories.

You might also find, for example, that you can't eat enough during the five to six meals a day. In that case, you may want to increase the number of meals you have each day to six to eight.

You must do *what it takes* to provide your body with the number of calories you need to start gaining weight, whether you need just five meals or eight meals a day.

How Much Should You Eat at Once?

How much food should you eat at each meal? When you are first getting used to solid foods again, chances are that you will only be eating relatively small amounts until you feel as though you can handle more food.

During this time, you will be losing even more weight. You want to start eating regularly, and increasing the amount of food that you eat, and you want to do it as soon as you are physically able to do so and hold the food down. The time that it takes to get there depends on the individual.

Naturally, the amount you will be able to eat at once depends on a number of different things, including your procedure as well as where you are in the healing process.

A big consideration is ratios. Most of the time, you will want protein as the highest part of your intake ratio. Having between one to three ounces of meat or other protein per meal is generally a good figure to keep in mind. You could have one to two eggs for a meal, a cup of plain yogurt or one to two teaspoons of peanut butter.

You will use other foods mentioned in the previous chapter to supplement the protein, which is the focus of the diet for most people.

Again, *everyone is different*. This means the exact amount that each person can handle will differ. In general, it is a good idea to eat until you feel full and only until you are full. You do not want to eat to the point where it causes pain. Again, remember to eat slowly so your brain can keep up with the state of your stomach's fullness.

Beverages

When it comes to beverages, you will generally want to have between eight and ten cups a day. This ensures you have enough liquid to help with digestion, as well as enough to keep hydrated. Since you have a smaller capacity now, dehydration can be a danger if you aren't careful.

Instead of having your beverages when you have your meals, you should have drinks between meals. Have them about twenty minutes to half an hour after you eat your meal.

How Many Calories Do You Need?

One of the other questions you will have is just how many calories you need to eat. When you are trying to retain your weight, you will generally want to have as many calories as possible in your diet. Once you are at a healthy weight, you need to maintain that weight.

Determining the actual amount of calories you need happens

on an individual basis. Based on your size, your weight, and your metabolism, you may need to have more or fewer calories than others will need. You will not find a "hard and true" number that will be true for everyone.

It takes time, adjustment, experimenting, and working with health professionals who can make sure you are getting the proper number of calories each day.

Carry Food with You and Think About Calories

You always want to have some food with you just in case you are out when it comes time to eat. Having some snacks that are easily portable and that you can eat while on the go is always a good idea. I will cover some good snack ideas later in the book, and you probably have a few of your favorites that are still good to eat as well. Just try to stay away from the sweet snacks.

You also want to get into the mindset where you are always looking for ways that you can add calories to your food. Consider ways that you can put even just a few extra calories into every meal. If you can add some butter or oil, bacon bits, a sauce, or some gravy, consider doing it. When you are trying to heal and gain weight, every single calorie counts!

How Do Your Feelings Affect Your Ability to Eat – The Psychology Behind Eating After Gastrectomy

Psychology can play a rather significant role in how you do after you go through surgery for your gastrectomy. It's natural for people to have a wide range of unpleasant feelings going through them when they are going through treatment and after their surgical procedure.

Some of the most common types of feelings include:

- Fear
- Anxiousness
- Depression
- Anger
- Helplessness

These feelings persist, and they can sometimes make it difficult to get onto a good eating plan, simply because your mind has trouble focusing.

Coping with these feelings can be difficult, but you must if you hope to get on an eating plan that will help to make you healthy again.

Tips for Feeling Better and Getting Your Weight Gain Plan Back on Track

Here is a short and effective list of tips that can help you when you are feeling down and when you feel like you just don't want to eat.

- **Talk** with someone you trust about what you are going through. While the person might not know exactly how you feel or why it can be so hard to eat – something they find easy – he or she will at least be able to listen to you and be there for you.

- **Meditation** is another method that some people use when they are trying to calm down and get a better sense of things. While it might not be the answer for everyone, it couldn't hurt to try it. Meditation in the morning before your first meal could be a good way to start the day off on the right foot.

- You may also find that joining a **cancer support group** for people going through things very similar to you can be helpful, as well. These are people who know and who understand just what it is you are going through. They've been there, and they are still there right now, just as you are.

- Something else that some people do is **make a list of foods** that they love and that they can still have on their new dietary lifestyle. Thinking about these foods, and making sure you have them in the pantry, helps some people to build up their appetite in anticipation of foods they love.
- Another thing you will want to do is to make sure you have plenty of **rest**. Getting at least seven to eight hours of sleep each day will make a big difference.
- You need your rest, but you should also try to be active as soon as you are physically capable. Once you have the clearance for some **light exercise**, do it. It will help you to feel better mentally and physically, and it can help to boost your appetite so you actually do feel like eating.

Meal Plan Sample

Here's a sample meal plan on a typical day for someone recovering from surgery and getting his or her eating back on track. This is just a sample, and not something you need to follow identically. Take this model, as well as the recipes that follow, and your own recipes, and then create your own plans.

In Chapter 11, I'll cover the steps you should take when you are putting together your plan.

Meal Plan
- Breakfast
  - o 1 scrambled egg
  - o 1 slice of whole grain toast, buttered
  - o ½ banana, mashed
  - o Drink ½ to 1 cup of milk about 20 minutes to half an hour after eating breakfast.

- Snack
  - 1 ounce cottage cheese or plain yogurt
  - 4 plain crackers
- Lunch
  - 2 ounces tuna fish with mayonnaise for sandwich
  - 2 slices whole grain bread
  - ½ sliced apple
  - ½ cup of fruit juice, about 20 minutes to half an hour after eating lunch
- Snack
  - 3 crackers
  - Peanut butter
  - 1 cup of water or fruit juice about 20 minutes to half an hour after snack
- Dinner
  - 2 ounces of protein (chicken or beef)
  - ½ cup mashed potatoes, with butter
  - ½ cup peas
  - ½ cup applesauce, unsweetened, for dessert
  - 1 cup of milk about 30 minutes after eating
- Snack
  - 3 slices of deli meat, such as turkey breast
  - Mayonnaise, spread onto the turkey, which you can then roll up
  - 1 cup of milk half an hour to an hour after eating

Make sure that you eat your last meal/snack early enough in the evening that you don't have to worry about any indigestion when you lay down to go to bed. Try to eat your last bit of food at least an hour or two before you have to go to bed, and you should not have any issues with this.

Summary

While the guidelines in this chapter should help you quite a bit when you are trying to determine just how much you should be eating and when you should eat, you will want to experiment and adjust your schedule as needed.

The sample meal plan should give you a good idea of about how much you should be eating each day, on average. Of course, people of different weights, and who may be trying to regain weight rather than maintain it may need to eat a bit more or less food, depending on their situation.

I have covered the best methods for how long you should wait between meals and how you should spread them throughout the day. Ultimately, though, you will want to listen to your own body and your doctor, dietician or nutritionist to create the plan that works the best for your specific needs.

CHAPTER 5

Gastrectomy Complications and Resolutions

After you have your gastrectomy, you may face a number of other complications. Some people will not have any of these issues, and others may have several problems. It's important to look into these various health problems so you will have a better idea of exactly what they are and what you may expect, as well as how you can deal with those issues.

Naturally, whenever you find you are having issues with your health and have any type of complication, the *first* thing you need to do is to make sure you get in contact with your healthcare professional right away.

The following are some of the most common issues that people face after undergoing a gastrectomy. You should always make note of these and any other symptoms you have in your food diary. This way, you will have a much better idea of exactly what type of foods and eating habits might be causing the problems.

Additional Unintended Weight Loss

While you are going through your cancer treatment, as well as the buildup to and immediately after the gastrectomy, you will lose a substantial amount of weight. When you have a partial stomach or no stomach after the procedure, it makes it even more difficult to keep on weight because of your reduced capacity.

The entirety of this book is to help you fight against this problem and the additional weight loss that can occur because of these other issues and health problems that might arise after the surgery.

Dumping Syndrome

Dumping syndrome is actually a group of symptoms some-times faced by those who have undergone a gastrectomy. What happens, at its most basic level, is that the contents in your stomach that are not yet digested move from your stomach and into the small bowel, which can cause a number of complications and is-sues.

Those who suffer from this problem generally find that it hap-pens very soon after eating. However, with others, it could take one, or even up to three hours before the symptoms occur. Some people actually have problems right after eating, and later in the digestive process.

What Are the Symptoms?

Dumping syndrome has a number of different symptoms, and they can vary based on how soon after eating one begins to feel them.

Those who have issues immediately after eating will have some of the following symptoms:

- Nausea
- Vomiting
- Diarrhea
- Uncomfortable feeling of fullness
- Abdominal cramps
- Dizziness
- Increased heart rate
- Flushed skin

For those who tend to develop symptoms later, the condition can include some or all of the following symptoms:

- Fatigue
- Sweating
- Hunger
- Increased heart rate
- Fainting
- Dizziness
- Confusion

One of the things that can cause dumping syndrome to be even worse is to have a meal high in sugar. This includes sucrose, or normal table sugar, and fructose, fruit sugar. If you notice that eating certain types of food causes this to happen with you, cut those out of your diet and replace them with better options. In the chapter on creating a food diary, I will discuss a bit more about how to monitor your intake.

Severe Complications Can Occur

If you start to notice these symptoms, and if changing your diet doesn't do anything to control them, then immediately see your doctor. Dumping syndrome could cause you to lose even more weight if you let it go unchecked, and this is highly dangerous to your health.

Sometimes, having low blood sugar can actually be a part of dumping syndrome, and your doctor may want to measure your blood sugar level during the time of your symptoms. This can aid in the diagnosis, and it may help them determine what you may need to add to your diet to help solve the problem.

Puzzlingly, having too little sugar in the body can cause the problem, as can having too much sugar.

Because of the symptoms surrounding dumping syndrome, some people actually end up developing a fear of eating. They do not want to have to deal with the discomfort that comes with the syndrome, so they stop eating. This leads to more weight loss.

Some people even find that the syndrome leads to a diminished social life and perhaps even anxiety and/or depression. They fear being away from home and away from the toilet. This can also make it difficult for some to keep their jobs when they are dealing with this problem chronically.

Treating the Problem

Most of the time, making changes to your diet and simply seeing how eating different foods and in different amounts can help you will improve the digestive process. Many people find that with the right diet and the right eating habits, they are able to eliminate dumping syndrome. Others are not quite so lucky though, and they may need to seek medical help.

Your doctor might prescribe medications that help to slow the digestive process in some cases. Some of the most common medications used are acarbose as a tablet and octreotide as an injection. Doctors only use these in the most severe circumstances, as slowing the digestive process too much means you will not absorb as many calories and nutrients as you need through the day, since you will not be able to eat as much. Some of the medications in use also have their own side effects, so your doctor is not going to want to prescribe them unless it is the *only* option.

Tips for Dealing with Dumping Syndrome

You will find that much of the advice given throughout this book is *already* aimed at helping you prevent dumping syndrome. Specialists, like myself, normally recommend that you change your diet and eat smaller meals, which you should already be doing. Most also advise avoiding fluids with your meals, as well as waiting for about half an hour after eating before having anything to drink.

Always chew your food completely and thoroughly before you swallow, as this helps to make digestion much easier. Also, make sure you have enough fiber and protein in your diet. Avoid drinking any alcohol, and be sure to stay away from acidic and spicy foods. Citrus fruits, tomatoes, and other foods that have high amounts of acid in them can be difficult for some to digest properly and can cause issues with you digestion.

When preparing your food, it's best to grill, bake, or broil. Avoid frying and similar methods of cooking, as it increases unhealthy fat and oils, which can cause issues with your digestive process. You want the calories, but you don't want to do anything that will cause dumping syndrome.

Finally, relax after eating and even lean back a bit. Slow things down a bit, so you can slow the movement of your food and so your body can rest during the digestive process.

Reflux Esophagitis

Another issue that can plague some who have gone through a gastrectomy is reflux esophagitis. This can cause irritation as well as inflammation in the esophagus, which can, in turn, make you have a number of different issues, including the following:

- Painful swallowing
- Sore throat
- Heartburn
- Sour or bitter taste in the mouth

This issue often occurs when you eat different types of foods, so it really is essential that you keep a good food diary and note the times you are eating, as well as the times of the symptoms. This should let you determine the culprit food more easily so you can eliminate it from your diet.

If the issue persists, and you can do nothing to remedy it on your own, you should speak with a doctor. Reflux can make it very difficult to absorb the nutrients you need. Some people who suffer from this problem tend to eat less as well because they do not want to deal with the pain and issues reflux causes.

How to Deal with the Problem?

One of the things you will find is that certain types of food tend to cause this problem. Caffeine, greasy foods, and peppermint are common causes, but they are not the only ones. You may find that you simply can't tolerate some type of foods without running into this issue.

In addition to eating more frequent but smaller meals through-out the day, as you should already be doing, and in addition to

48

eliminating certain foods, you have some other options to help with the issue as well. Consider wearing looser clothing so there is less pressure on your abdominal area, for example.

If you still have issues, speak with a doctor about medications he or she may be able to prescribe for you. Deal with the problem as soon as you can so you don't have to worry about missing calories and losing more weight.

Loss of Appetite

Loss of appetite can happen for any number of reasons. It could be related to the cancer and the treatment, pain, fatigue, and the sheer stress of trying to deal with everything.

Anxiety and depression are common for many people. This is particularly true in the immediate aftermath of the surgery, and for several months after.

One of the ways to deal with the loss of appetite is to "graze or nibble" throughout the day. Perhaps you don't feel hungry enough to eat on a schedule. To make sure you are still getting the nutrients you need, consider eating throughout the day whenever you have the chance. You can slowly work your way toward a regular schedule.

Also, try your best to relax and focus on positive things when it is mealtime. Health experts often say that you shouldn't watch television while you eat because you may eat more than you realize. This is actually perfect for those who are trying to get enough calories in the day! Consider putting on one of your favorite shows and simply getting lost in it while you eat your meals.

You should also be careful how you are taking your liquids. Most people are used to drinking with their meals. This is simply the way most people have always done things. I've mentioned it before, but it bears repeating. Don't drink your fluids with your meals. It makes you feel full too fast and reduces your appetite. Drink between meals instead.

Changes in Taste or Sense of Smell

One of the other things that you might notice is that foods may taste and smell different. Some people complain that meat, for example, tastes bitter, or that it has a metallic taste. Foods you once loved the smell of may now make you feel nauseous, too.

A number of different things, from your cancer to the treatment, and even dental health issues, can cause these changes to occur. While there is no real way to treat these issues, most find that they will eventually diminish. The hard part is actually learning to love to eat again *while* you are dealing with the issue.

Tips for Dealing with Changes in Taste and Smell

It is now time for some experimentation. You will want to find foods that still appeal to your sense of smell and your taste and avoid the ones that you no longer like. For example, you may no longer be able to stand the smell of cooking fish, or you may not like the taste. If that's the case, simply move on to another protein, such as turkey or chicken.

Make the foods taste a bit different, too. For example, you can use herbs and simple spices to add some flavor. Oregano, basil, and rosemary are typically good choices, but you have a number of great options. Marinades can also work quite well. Experiment to find the ones that you like and can tolerate the best.

Another tip that has worked for some people who complain of a metal taste in their mouth while eating is to use plastic utensils rather than metal. Some have also started cooking their food in glass pots and pans, too.

Dry Mouth

Dry mouth is another issue some have after a gastrectomy. Having less saliva can present you with a number of difficulties. It can make it harder to speak, chew, and even swallow your food.

Interestingly, this links with the last problem as well, as some complain that a dry mouth changes the way their food tastes, not to mention the enjoyment of the food.

Why Does This Happen?

You may suffer from dry mouth for a variety of reasons. The treatments you've undergone and the medicines you are taking may be the culprits. Fortunately, you can do some things that can correct this problem.

Tips for Helping with Dry Mouth

First, consider sipping water throughout the day to keep your saliva levels higher. This helps you swallow and talk. Just don't drink *with* your meals. You can also chew some sugarless gum or have some sugarless hard candy, which can help generate more saliva in your mouth. Some choose to have some tart foods, which help them to make more saliva.

Lactose Intolerance

Being lactose intolerant means that your body no longer has the ability to absorb and digest lactose, a sugar in milk and milk products. The symptoms can vary, and often include cramps and gas,; eating these types of foods – cheese, milk, and ice cream – that in lactose intolerance can be very unpleasant indeed.

This can be especially problematic for someone who has had a gastrectomy and trying to increase weight, as milk and similar products are a part of the diet for most people.

How to Deal With Lactose Intolerance

Look for lactose-free substitutes out there. Most of the time, you should be able to find alternates in the grocery store that are free of lactose, or that have only a small amount of the sugar in them.

Some of the best alternatives are soy milk, almond milk, coconut and rice milk. Please keep in mind that these *do taste different.* However, they have a pleasant taste, and you should be able to get used to them. Just make sure that soy and these other ingredients are agreeable with you before you invest too heavily in using them. Try different brands or some with vanilla for added flavor.

Having lactose intolerance can make it more difficult when it comes to eating out and eating at a friend's house. If you are lactose intolerant, you should make sure that you are very careful about knowing exactly what is in the food you eat so you do not have any painful or gaseous surprises.

Constipation

Medications, lack of fiber, and many other things can cause constipation, and if you are suffering from this, you know it is not pleasant. Thankfully, here are some simple remedies that should be able to work most of the time.

First, make sure you have plenty of liquids throughout the day. This can be hard if you have had a gastrectomy, as you should only be drinking between meals. Make it a point to get plenty of fluid though to prevent constipation, dehydration, and dry mouth. Keep a water bottle handy for quick access. Have hot liquids in your diet as well, such as tea or even soup broth.

Eating high fiber foods can be helpful as well. If you are eating the whole grains we talked about earlier, they can help quite a bit. Just make sure you are not overdoing it with the fiber, as it makes you feel full faster, and that leads to less of an intake of calories and nutrients.

It's all about balancing.

Diarrhea

If you are suffering from diarrhea, then it can be a very dangerous scenario. This means that food may be moving through your system too fast and you may not be absorbing all of the nutrients that you should, which will lead to other health issues. This can happen for a number of reasons, including some cancer treatments and medicine, as well as diet.

Tips for Dealing with Diarrhea

Make sure you have plenty of fluids in your system, as you will be going through liquids very quickly when you suffer from this issue. You need to replace those fluids. Of course, you also need to make sure you are not drinking so much water that you are no longer hungry.

Look for some foods that are higher in sodium and potassium, so you can replenish these elements in your body. Consider eating some low fiber foods as well. Have your drinks at room temperature, and avoid foods and drinks that can actually exacerbate the problem. Again, it's all about finding out what your body can and cannot handle.

Some of the foods you will want to avoid if you are suffering from diarrhea include:

- Pasta
- Sugary drinks – which you should be avoiding anyway
- Hot or cold drinks
- Fried and greasy food
- Raw fruits and vegetables that cause you to have gas
- Milk products
- Caffeinated drinks
- Spicy food
- Products that contain sorbitol or xylitol, which are artificial sweeteners
- Apple juice, which is often high in sorbitol

Nausea

Some people have feelings of unease and queasiness, and sometimes they may even feel the need to vomit. In some cases, they will actually vomit, but that does not always happen. As with most of these health issues, a number of things can cause the problem, including the smell of food.

The best way to deal with this problem is to eat foods that are easy on your stomach and that do not have unpleasant smells. Snacking on dry toast or crackers to help settle the stomach can help as well.

You might discover that you feel nauseous only at certain times of the day, such as the morning. Note the times when you have these feelings; then, incorporate these issues in to your eating plan so you can eat when your body feels best able to deal with eating.

Sore Mouth

People who suffer from a sore mouth, possibly due to the therapy they've undergone or because of dental problems, will find that eating can be difficult.

Those who are suffering from this problem will want to choose foods that are easy to chew and that they can cut into small pieces, or even puree if needed. Cook the foods until they are nice and tender, and even use smaller utensils so you do not have to open your mouth as far. Some even choose to use a straw to drink their liquids, as it is easier on their mouth.

Naturally, you will want to avoid certain types of foods when you have a sore mouth as well. These include:

- Citrus fruits and juices
- Anything spicy
- Salty foods
- Raw vegetables
- Sharp or crunchy foods

Food Care and Preparation Tips

Something else you will need to consider with your new diet, particularly in the early months after the surgery, is ensuring you do not contract any infections. Preparing and handling your food the right way reduces the risk of food-borne infections. Here are some very simple tips to avoid food-borne infections:

- Make sure you keep leftovers refrigerated, and put them in the fridge as soon as you finish eating. Make sure you scrub all of your fruits and veggies before you eat them, and if you can't wash the foods well, then avoid them.

- Always wash your countertop, hands, and knives that you use before and after you use them. This is especially important when you are preparing meats and fish. Have two cutting boards as well – one for your vegetables and fruit and one for your fish. Make sure they are different enough in color or material that you do not confuse the two.

- Cook meats completely. The meat should not have any pink inside, and consider using a meat thermometer to check internal temperature. Even if you like rare steak, cook them thoroughly. After the procedure you've undergone, you can't afford a sickness or infection.

- Some other good tips include not eating raw fish, making sure you buy pasteurized products, and if you are going out to eat, stay away from buffets, which could be crawling with bacteria and infections.

Summary

These are some of the most common health complications and problems people who have undergone a gastrectomy may have to face. While not all individuals have these problems, now that you know how to deal with them, you can rest easy knowing you can face and defeat any and all of the complications that might arise.

If you have these or other issues that are simply too problematic to handle on your own, you will naturally want to make sure you get to the doctor as soon as you can.

CHAPTER 6

Breakfast Recipes

When you first wake up in the morning, you might not feel like eating immediately, and it might be an hour or two before you really feel as though you can eat and hold down food. Others find that they can eat right away, almost as soon as they roll out of the bed in the morning.

One of the things you will note with the breakfast recipes I've included in this book is that they are relatively simple. I'm keeping them simple on purpose, so you can start with the best basic, tasty foods out there, and then add to it as you learn which other types of foods your body is able to tolerate.

Creating complex recipes that have items that don't agree with you will not do you much good at all! Simple is better in the beginning, so you can take the basics and then create your own special recipes from them.

Now, let's get on to some breakfast favorites!

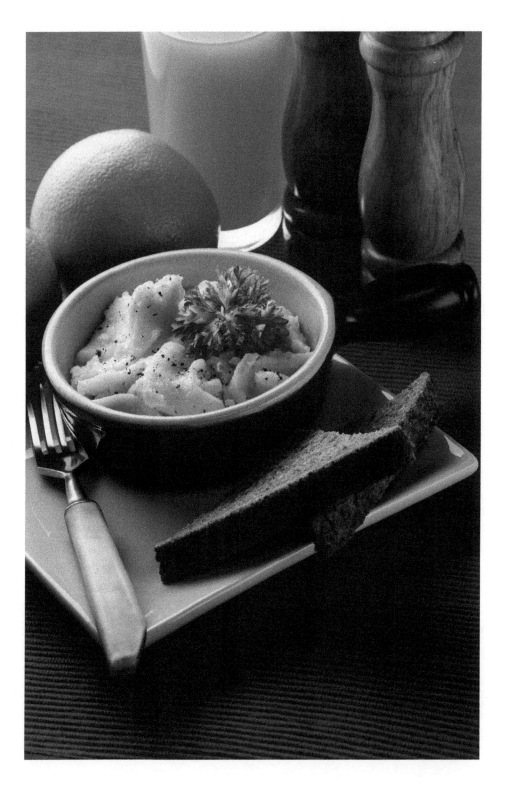

Simple Scrambled Eggs

Scrambled eggs are a staple of breakfast, but some people still have trouble making them properly. They are not overly difficult, but it does take some practice to get them just right. Fortunately, the practice can be quite tasty. The secret is in the cream.

Ingredients:
- 1 to 2 eggs
- Salt and pepper
- 1 T of butter, unsalted
- 1 T of heavy cream

Crack the eggs into a bowl, add about a pinch of salt and pepper to the bowl and then whisk the eggs until thoroughly mixed.

In a small saucepan, add butter and turn the heat on to medium. Once the butter melts and coats the bottom of the pan, pour in the eggs. Begin whisking and fluffing them right away. Keep whisking as they are cooking, and then remove them from the heat, finally adding your cream to the mix and stirring it into the eggs.

Now, it's ready to serve along with some toast or fruit. The addition of the cream is a nice and easy way to add some more calories.

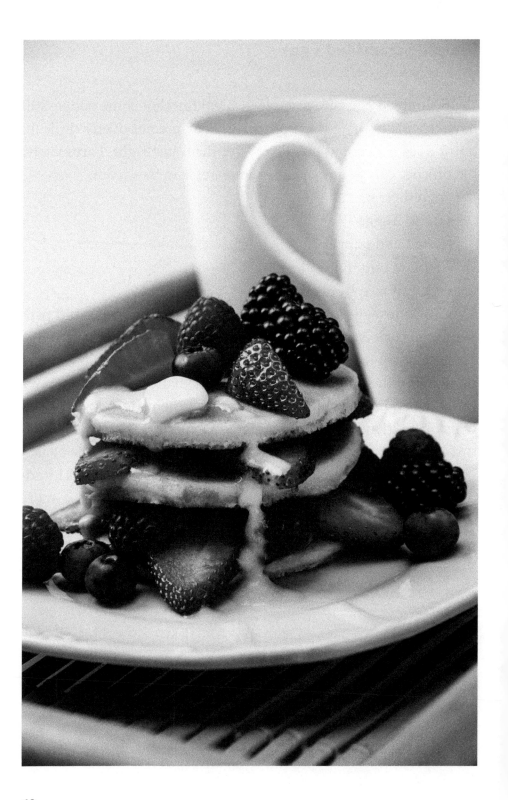

Whole Grain Pancakes

Pancakes are another important part of breakfast, and just because you are not going to be eating any sweets on this diet, it does not mean that you have to give up pancakes. Instead, just start buying some whole grain pancake mix, which has a surprisingly good taste.

You can also make them on your own without a mix, although it does take a bit more effort. Here's an easy recipe to get you started.

Ingredients:

- 1 cup milk
- 1 T vinegar
- 1 cup whole wheat flour
- 2 tsp artificial sweetener
- ½ tsp baking powder
- ¼ tsp baking soda
- ¼ tsp salt
- 1 egg
- 2 T butter, melted, plus additional butter for the griddle

Mix wet ingredients in one bowl and dry ingredients in another bowl. Preheat a nonstick griddle to 375 degrees or gas mark 5, and then mix your wet and dry ingredients together. Mix them so that there is no flour remaining, but keep the lumps, as this will ensure they are nice and fluffy rather than chewy. Not taking out all of the lumps from homemade or store bought mixes is why they often come out with a chewy texture!

Use an ice cream scooper to scoop out the mix onto the griddle. Cook until they start to bubble, then flip them with a spatula and continue cooking until the bottom side is nice and golden brown.

Serve with some additional butter and fresh fruit, but avoid syrup unless you have a sugar free variety.

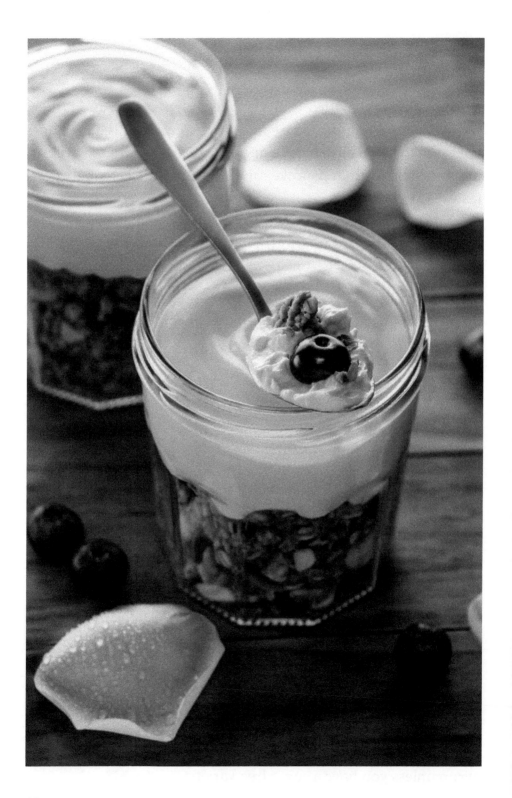

Fast and Easy Breakfast Parfait

Here's a quick and very simple breakfast recipe that tastes great. You don't just have to eat it at breakfast, either, as it can make a great snack just about any time of day when you want to get in a few more calories.

Ingredients:

- ½ cup plain or sugar free yogurt
- ¼ cup cereal –your choice of brand, but stay away from sweetened cereals
- ¼ cup fresh fruit

In a dish or a glass, layer these three ingredients, yogurt, cereal, and then another layer of yogurt. Follow this with a fruit layer and then with another layer of yogurt. Repeat until you've used all of the ingredients. Chill for about twenty minutes to an hour. If you don't eat it all at once, don't worry. It will keep in the refrigerator throughout the day, so you can come back and snack at your leisure!

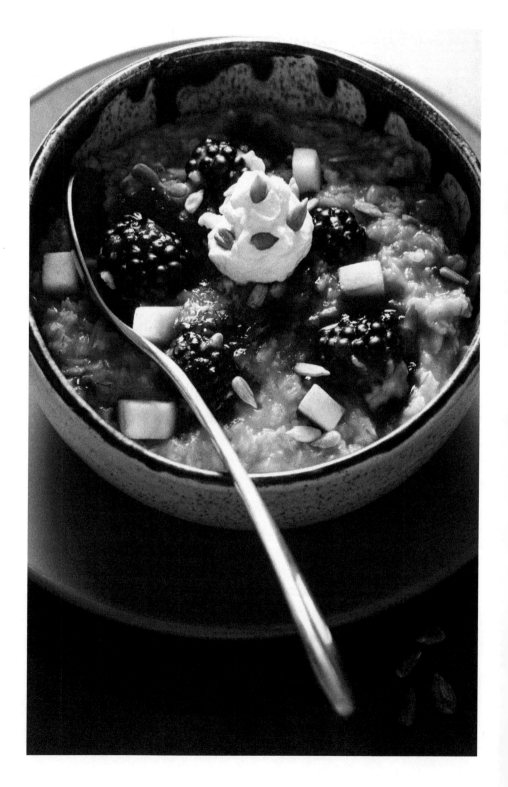

Oatmeal 2.0

Oatmeal can be good for you, but it tends to fill you up very quickly and sit in your stomach. You should make sure you are getting as many calories as possible when you have your oatmeal in the morning, so here is a nice 2.0 recipe to help!

Ingredients:

- 1 cup oatmeal
- ¼ cup blueberries, or fruit of your choice
- 1 tsp sunflower seeds

Cook your oatmeal according to the instructions – instant or traditional – and then simply add the seeds and the blueberries. If you would like to add a few more extra calories, you could even add a tablespoon of cream to the mix!

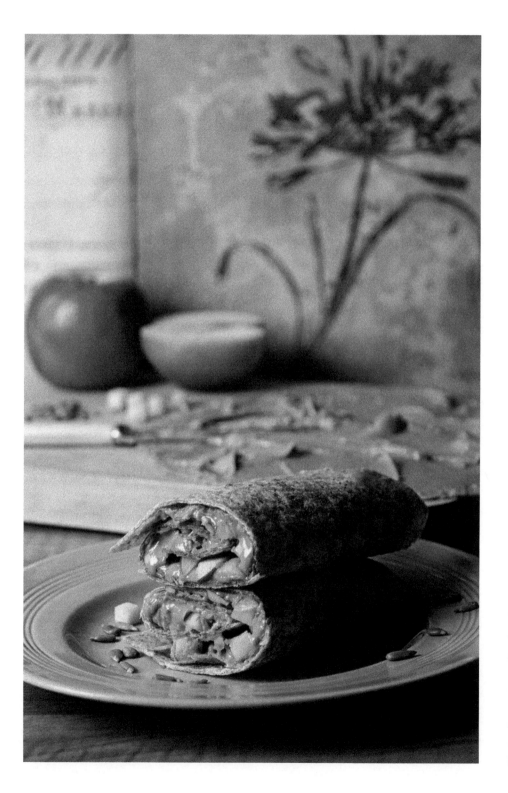

Peanut Butter Breakfast Wrap

Here's a nice and simple wrap that tastes great in the morning, and it has plenty of calories and nutrients to get you started off right. You might find this recipe to be another one that could work for a snack throughout the day.

Ingredients:
- 1 whole wheat wrap/tortilla
- 1 -2 tsp peanut butter
- Apple slices, your choice
- 1 tsp oats or sunflower seeds

Spread the peanut butter onto the tortilla and then sprinkle the seeds or oats onto it. Top it with the apple slices, then roll up the tortilla and enjoy!

Another option is to warm the tortilla in the microwave after, or even before, adding the peanut butter. If you put it in the microwave, it should only be in there for about ten to twenty seconds.

Summary

These are just five of the many different breakfast recipes out there you will be able to enjoy on your new diet. As delicious as these recipes sound, they don't have any table sugar in them, they are full of calories and protein, and they really do taste fantastic.

Try these out soon!

CHAPTER 7

Lunch Recipes

Now it's time for some lunch recipes! Keep in mind that even though I've divided these recipes into different sections for breakfast, lunch, dinner, and snacks, that doesn't mean you have to stick to eating them at certain times of the day.

Do whatever is right for you and for your diet plan. Eat what you want when you want, as long as you are getting enough calories and nutrients throughout the day. Again, I'm keeping these relatively easy to make and easy to adjust to suit your tastes.

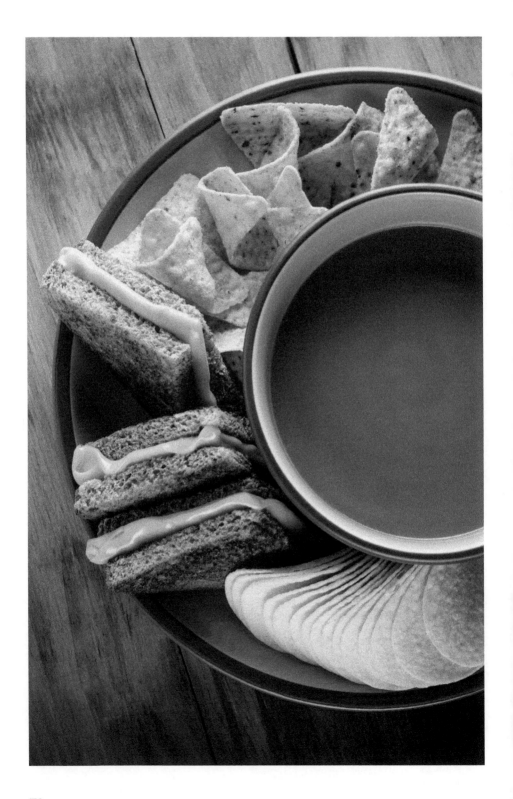

Easy Grilled Cheese

Everyone loves grilled cheese. The sandwiches have a fast and easy lunch recipe that you could pair with a bit of hearty soup, some chips, or any other high calorie goodie, too.

Ingredients:

- 2 slices whole grain bread
- 1 slice cheese
- 1 T butter, with additional for skillet

Preheat a skillet on medium heat. Place some butter into the skillet, as well as butter on one side of the bread. Place the bread butter side down into the skillet. Let it start to cook and then add a slice of cheese. Then, butter one side of the remaining piece of bread. Place this on top of the cheese with the butter side facing up. Grill until it is a light brown color, flip and finish cooking.

If you are in a big hurry, and you can't afford to spend the time making an actual grilled cheese sandwich, you can make an alternate version. Simply use a toaster oven and foregoing the butter. It doesn't have the same authentic taste, but it is fast, and if you have trouble with having too much grease in your diet, this could be a good alternative.

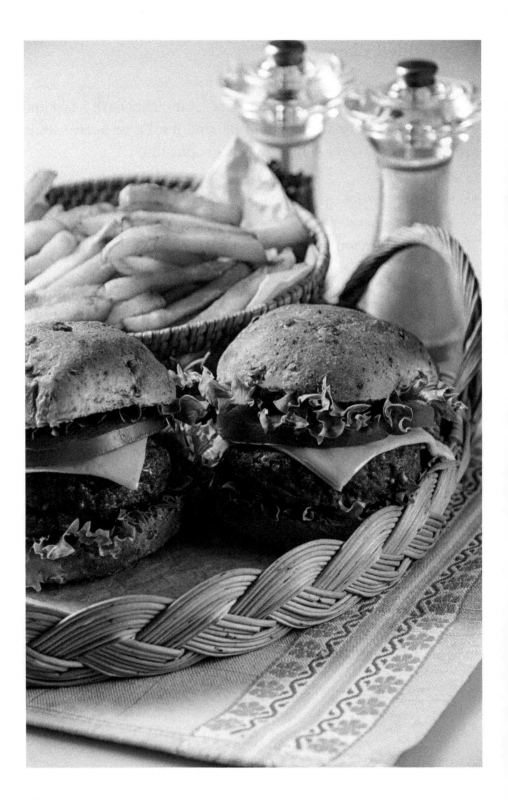

Cheeseburger and Chips

The hamburger and cheeseburger are classic, and when you make it at home, you can do it your way and have full control over how it tastes, as well as the ingredients you add.

Ingredients
- 2 ounces meat – ground beef or ground turkey
- 1 whole wheat bun
- 1 slice cheese, your choice
- Lettuce
- 1 T mayonnaise

This one's quite easy. Simply form the meat into a patty and put it onto a skillet, and then cook until it is done completely. Once it is nearly finished cooking, add the cheese to melt. Add your toppings and condiments, and serve with some chips or fries. A good trick to adding some more calories to fries is to serve them with gravy.

It can be fun to experiment and create your own "burger concoctions" as well. Consider adding some toppings that might not be traditional so you can add a bit of variety to your diet. This is where the fun comes into play! Some of the toppings you might want to consider for some added calories and taste include:

- Bacon
- Guacamole
- Pesto
- Sliced ham
- Avocado
- Fried egg
- Peanut butter

Avoid ketchup, which is high in sugar. Instead just add a sliced tomato.

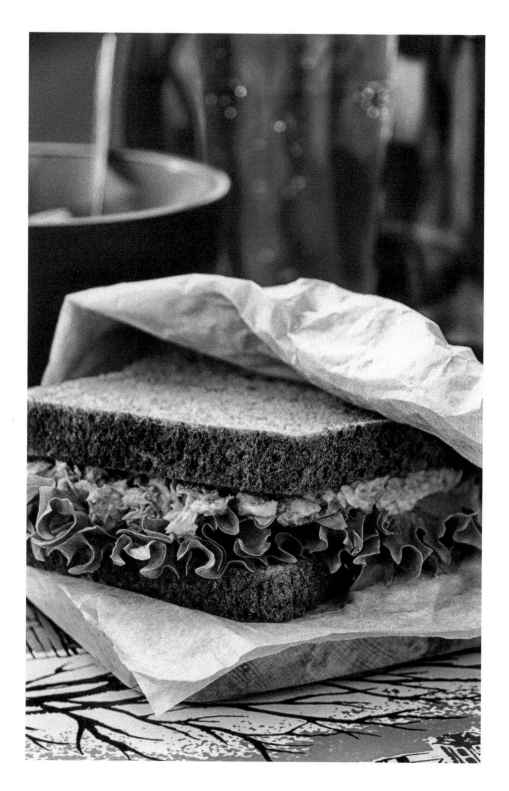

Terrific Tuna Sandwich

Tuna is fast and easy as well, and because of this it is one of the most popular lunch items. Of course, the delicious taste is another reason it is popular!

Ingredients:

- Canned tuna, packed in water or in oil
- 1-2 T mayonnaise
- Salt and pepper to taste
- 2 slices whole grain bread
- Leafy greens

Mix tuna and mayonnaise into a bowl; add your salt and pepper, and then add a spoonful or two to the bread. Spread it onto the bread, add lettuce or other leafy greens, and then cut it in half. If you prefer, use a whole wheat wrap rather than bread, and add other ingredients other than the greens, such as chopped pickles.

When use an entire can of tuna, you will likely have some leftover that you will not be able to eat in a single setting. Simply put it in a container, cover it, and put it in the fridge. You can bring it out later and put it on crackers for a tasty snack.

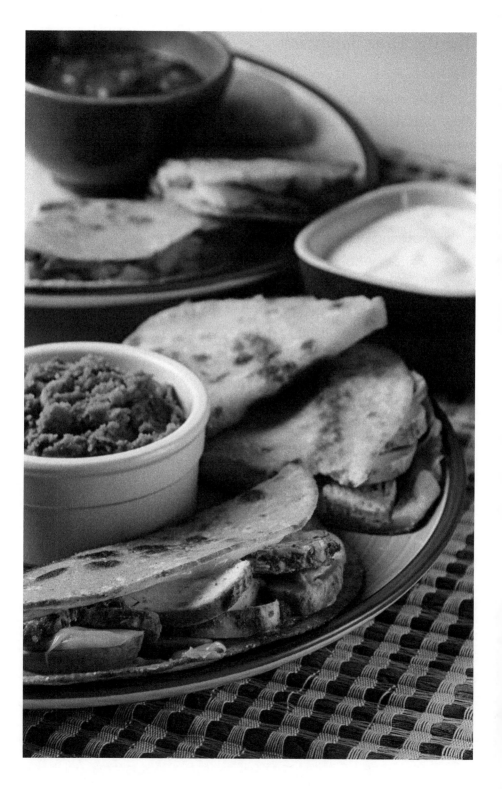

Quick Quesadillas

Quesadillas are tasty and they can be fun to make since you have so much variety in what will go into them. While this is a simple chicken and cheese recipe, you can alter the ingredients to suit your tastes.

Ingredients:

- 2 T butter
- 1 to 2 ounces sliced, cooked chicken breast
- 1 ounce of shredded cheese
- 2 slices avocado
- 1 ounce sour cream
- 1 whole wheat tortilla

Brush one side of the tortilla with butter and place it butter side down in the skillet. Add cheese, chicken, then avocado to the top one side of the tortilla, making sure to leave room to fold the tortilla without the ingredients toppling – it takes time to master this technique.

Fold it and cook it over medium heat for about three to four minutes on each side. Each side should be golden brown. Once it is done, take it out and serve with a side of sour cream. For some added calories, add a spoonful of refried beans on the side.

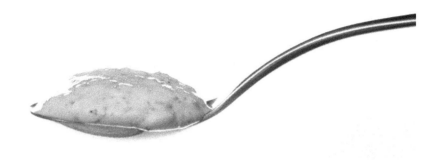

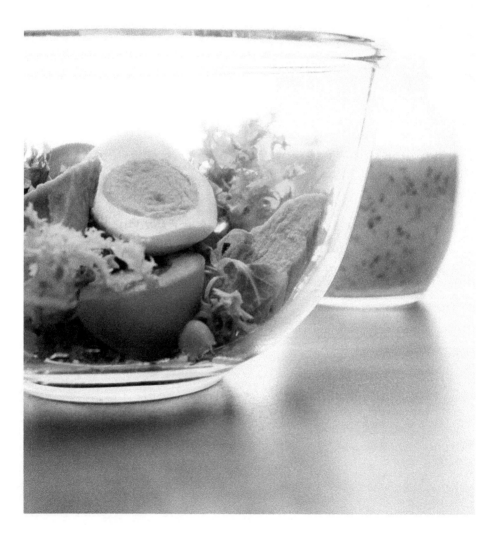

Big Salad

One of the issues with salad when you have had a gastrectomy is trying to gain weight. There are simply not enough calories in a traditional salad to be worth your while. That's why you shouldn't have a traditional salad. Instead, it's time to go big and add some ingredients.

Ingredients:

- Veggies – your choice of lettuce and other favorite vegetables
- 1 hardboiled egg
- Shredded cheese
- Sliced deli meat – ham and turkey
- Your choice of salad dressing – high calorie, but make sure it doesn't have added sugar

Mix your ingredients, and make sure to go heavier on the protein and lighter on the lettuce… something most people don't say when they are talking about a salad! This big salad has big protein and big calories, and it really can be a great meal. It also happens to be easy to make.

Summary

These are some fun and easy to make lunch recipes that you can take, renovate, and really make your own. Take the basics of these recipes and rework them until they are perfect for your taste buds.

CHAPTER 8

Dinner Recipes

Now it's time to move on to dinner recipes. Again, these are nice and easy, so you will be able to make them without spending too much time in the kitchen. The last thing you want to do is spend time preparing meals, so I've made these as simple as possible without sacrificing taste.

I have pared down the addition of spices and herbs, as you will want to add a few at a time as you learn about any changes to your food tolerances.

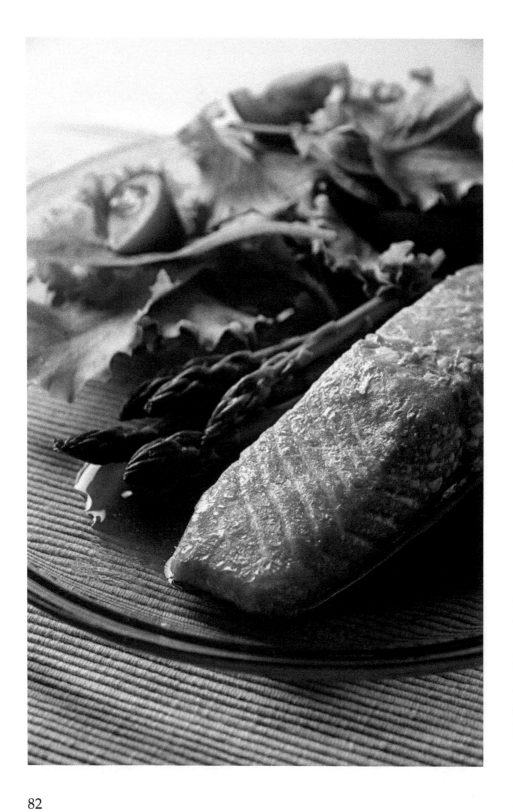

Broiled Fish and Veggies

Fish is an excellent source of protein, and it doesn't take very long to cook. Add to that that it tastes great, and it can make an ideal, quick dinner. It also feels very "light" despite all of the protein, so it is possible to get plenty of nutrients without ever feeling overly full.

Ingredients:

- Choices of fish steak – 1 to 2 ounces – salmon, tuna, and tilapia are some good options
- 2 T soy sauce
- 2 T unsweetened pineapple juice
- 1 T lemon juice, as long as you aren't overly sensitive to citrus
- Salt and pepper to taste
- Your choice of vegetables

Mix soy sauce, pineapple juice, lemon juice, and salt and pepper in a bowl to make marinade. Use this marinade to coat salmon or other fish, and then place it in a plastic bag. Pour the remaining juice into the bag, seal, and put into the refrigerator for about an hour or so.

Then, drain the marinade, and place the salmon in the oven in a sleeve of aluminum foil. You can also add your veggies to the foil, or you can cook them separately. Broil the fish for about twenty minutes. The result is a tasty fish thanks to a marinade that is not too sweet and not overpowering.

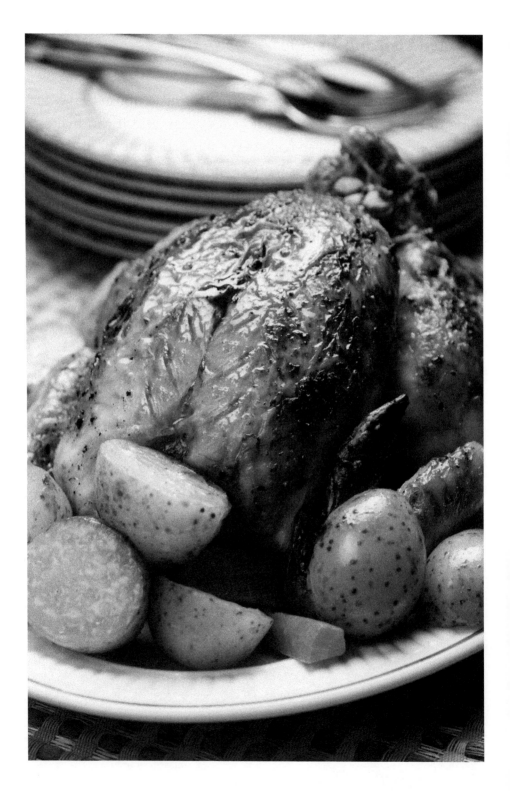

Roast Chicken and Potatoes and More

Roast chicken tastes great, it's healthy and full of protein, and it is extremely easy to cook. You can often find some great deals on roasting chickens in the store, too, so when you find a good price, buy a couple of them. They make for great leftovers, and you can even turn the leftover chicken into other interesting meals, such as chicken salad, chicken potpie, chicken soup and more.

Ingredients:

- 1 uncooked roasting chicken
- Potatoes – your choice of variety
- Carrots – cut into small chunks, or baby carrots
- 2 T olive oil
- Salt and pepper to taste

Preheat your oven to 375 degrees or gas mark 5. Place the chicken into a roasting pan. Rub it with the oil and the salt and pepper. If you do not want to use olive oil for this, you can use butter. It has more calories, and it can give the chicken a nice taste.

Add the vegetables to the roasting pan, along with about half a cup of water. Place it in an oven, covered, for about an hour to an hour and a half depending on the size of the chicken.

Make sure the chicken is cooked completely before taking it out by checking that the juices are no longer pink when you cut it. The vegetable should be nice and tender as well, as it makes them easier to chew and digest. Speaking of the veggies, you can add other types to the roast if you like. Just make sure you can handle eating them.

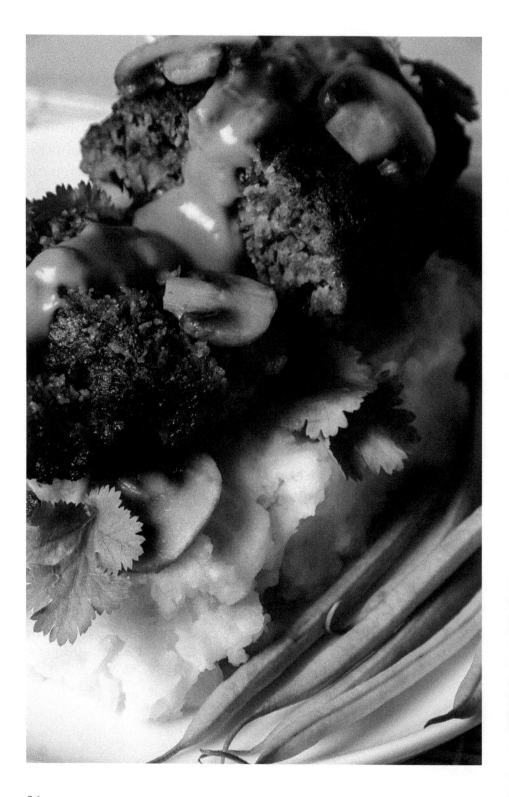

Meatloaf and Gravy

For many people, meatloaf is comfort food. It also has the potential to be very high in calories, not to mention delicious. These two elements are ones you certainly want from your meals!

Here's a very simple recipe for meatloaf and brown gravy you will want to try.

Ingredients:

- 1 ½ pounds ground beef
- ¾ cup bread crumbs – make sure to use whole grain bread crumbs
- 1 egg
- 1 cup mushrooms, sliced
- 1 T butter
- 1 cup beef broth
- 2 T water
- 1 T cornstarch
- Salt and pepper to taste

Preheat the oven to 350 degrees or gas mark 4.

Combine beef, egg, salt and pepper, and mix it well. Shape it into a loaf and place it in a pan. If you have a loaf pan, go ahead and use it. If you don't, the loaf should actually be stable enough to sit in a larger pan – even a cake pan if necessary. Bake in the oven for about an hour or meat is cooked through.

When you take the meatloaf out to cool, it's time to make this simple gravy, which will add loads of calories and taste. In a medium saucepan, melt butter on medium heat. Add the mushrooms and cook until tender. Then, add the beef broth and simmer for about five minutes. Stir occasionally.

Combine the cornstarch and the water into a small cup and then stir that mixture into the broth. It should only take about a minute or so until it thickens into a nice brown gravy.

Some good and tasty sides that will go along well with this meal might be mashed potatoes or green beans.

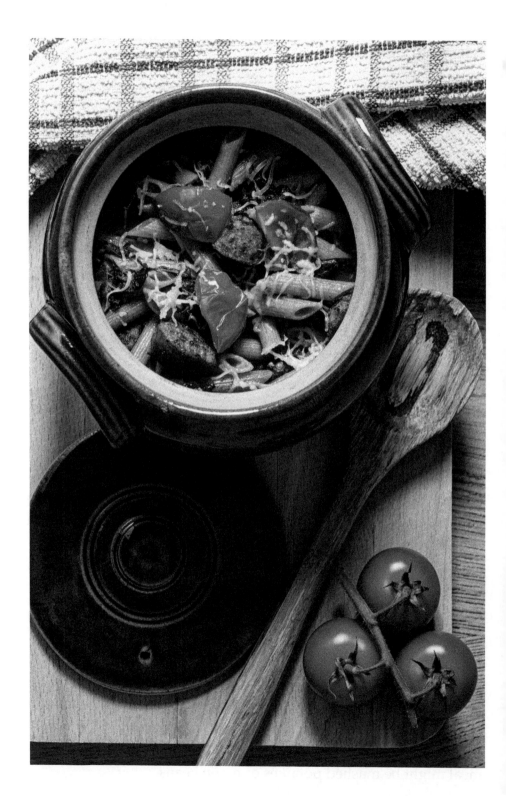

Whole Wheat Pasta and Sausage

Wheat pasta is surprisingly good, and it has a nice texture that will not make you miss the old pasta at all. Here's a nice and simple recipe that will give you that pasta you crave. One word of caution is with the sausage that you choose. Sausage is a great choice for protein and taste, but you will want to make sure you choose an option that is not spicy, as you might not be able to handle the spice.

Ingredients:

- ¾ pound of wheat pasta
- 1 pound of sausage
- 1 T olive oil
- 1 can chicken broth
- 1 package frozen spinach – ten ounces
- ½ cup parmesan cheese, grated

Bring pasta to a boil and cook for about eight to ten minutes, or until it has the perfect tenderness for your taste. It is easier to eat and digest when you avoid the al dente options with pasta, so keep that under consideration while cooking. Strain pasta and set aside.

Cook sausage in a skillet until it is done and no longer pink. During the last five to six minutes of cooking, add the broth and the spinach to the mixture. You can add tomatoes as well, but keep in mind that they are acidic and may not be an ideal option for everyone who has undergone a gastrectomy.

Finally, add the pasta to the mix, stir, add the cheese, and serve. It's fast, tasty, and another recipe where you can experiment with the ingredients until you find the ones that work the best for your taste buds.

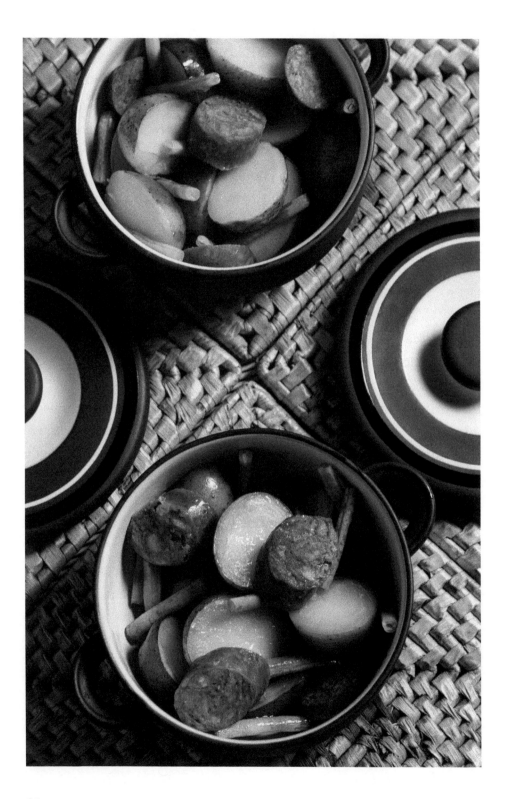

Smoked Sausage, Potato and Green Bean Mix

Here's another recipe for some delicious sausage. Again, experiment with the options out there to find out which ones you can eat without issue, and which ones you like the taste of the most.

Ingredients:

- ¾ pound green beans – fresh or frozen
- ½ pound red potatoes
- 1 pound smoked sausage
- Salt and pepper to taste
- 1 tsp olive oil
- 1/3 cup water

Preheat the oven to 375 or gas mark 5. Then, prepare your vegetables. Place aluminum foil into a large baking dish and add the potatoes, green beans, water, salt and pepper, and olive oil. Close the foil to make a pouch and leave just a small opening at the top. Place in the oven and cook until the vegetables are tender.

Cook sausage in a skillet until done. Many brands of smoked sausages actually come precooked, so the only thing you really need to do is reheat them. Make sure you read the packaging so you don't undercook sausage by mistake!

Combine the veggies and the sausage and serve.

Summary

These are some nice and easy to make dinners, and you will find that you will generally have plenty of leftovers when you make these recipes. Keep them in the fridge and you can eat them the next day for your lunch as well. It makes it easier to have meals ready to go as soon as you are hungry.

Another thing you will notice about the recipes in this book is that they are generally easy to reheat right in the microwave. Again, I'm trying to make things as easy as possible for you, while still providing the nutrition – and taste – you need.

Feel free to experiment a bit with these recipes as well. Add some ingredients that you like, and substitute ones that you don't. It's all about making the food appealing to your tastes and making the experience of eating as pleasant as possible for you.

Consider starting your own recipe book, and keeping it alongside your food diary. In time, you will have a great collection of recipes that suit your tastes perfectly.

CHAPTER 9

Drinks, and More

The beverages you consume are about more than just hydration, or at least they can be. While you certainly need to continue ingesting enough water to ensure you never feel dehydrated, you also want to find some ways to get a few extra calories and taste from your beverages. In this chapter, I will go over some of the ways that you can do just that.

In addition, I've included a couple of very simple to make sugar free marinade recipes. Use these when you are preparing meat and even vegetables to add a few more calories and a lot more taste.

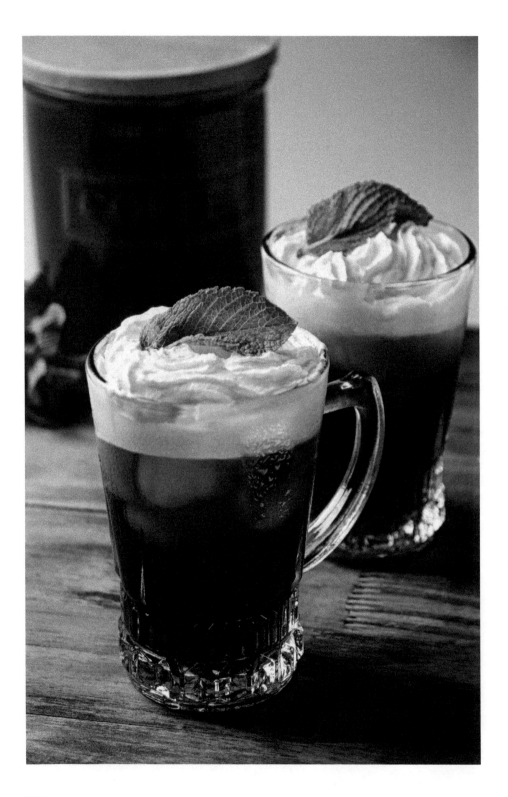

Iced Coffee

Who doesn't love iced coffee? Of course, most of us don't enjoy spending an arm and a leg at the coffee shop to get something that's full of sugar and has no real nutritional value. Fortunately, it's possible to make your own iced coffee for less money and with less sugar, and you will be able to do it quite easily.

Ingredients:

- Coffee
- Ice – or just the fridge
- Artificial sweeteners
- Sugar free creamer

This is quite simple and quite delicious. All you need to do is make coffee as you normally would, and then cool it down. You can wait until the pot is cool enough to put into the refrigerator and throw some ice cubes into it.

Use artificial sweeteners, or sugar free creamer to give the coffee a bit more of a sweet taste without actually adding any sugar. If you are lactose intolerant, you can find sugar free nondairy creamers you can use as well.

It's nice and easy, and a good way to wake up in the morning!

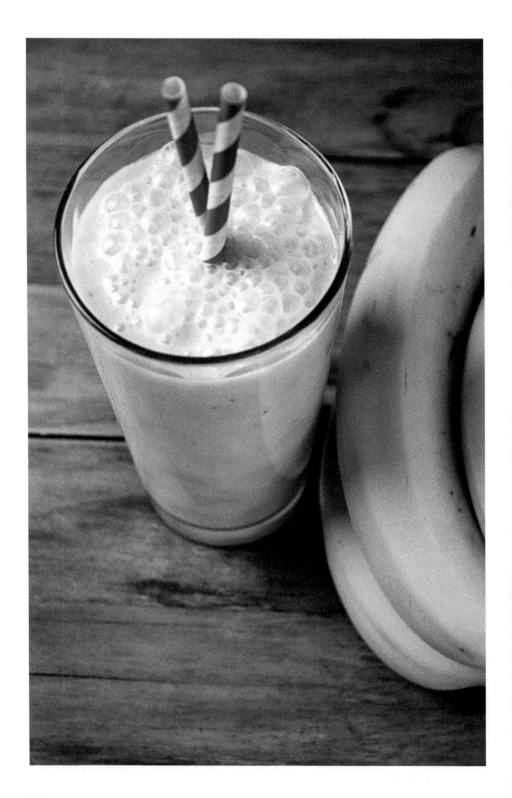

Banana Milk and Other Smoothie Drinks

Here's a good way to get some extra calories in your drinks. If you love the taste of bananas, you will go, well, *bananas* for this drink! It tastes great, is full of potassium, is easy to make, and there's even a way to add just a bit more protein to it to make it even better.

Ingredients:

- ½ banana, ripe
- ½ to 1 cup milk
- ½ T artificial sweetener
- 1 T protein powder
- ½ tsp vanilla extract

Simply put all of these ingredients into the blender and blend until nice and smooth. You could add a cube or two of ice if you want to make it taste a bit more like a smoothie. Easy, delicious, and nutritious!

There are countless smoothie options out there, and to go through all of them would be impossible, especially given the fact that everyone's tastes are different.

Peanut butter is also a very good ingredient choice, and it is just packed with protein. You can even add some sugarless jelly to the smoothie for a PB&J! Smoothie recipes are actually very easy and very fun to create on your own, so have a good time experimenting with all different types of fruit.

Just make sure to start off with simple mixes with just a few ingredients. This way you can test to see if your body can handle the ingredients before adding to it.

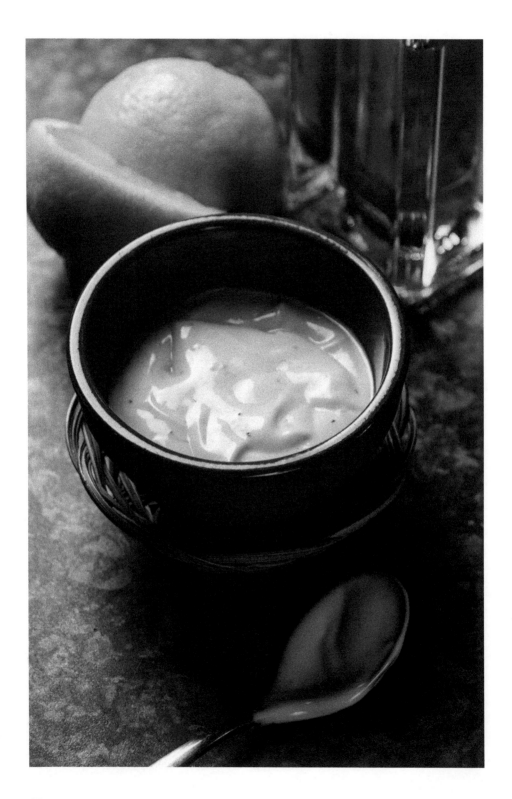

Marinade #1

Here's a nice recipe for a marinade that should be able to give you some added zing and calories to your meals without any added sugar. It's easy to make and tastes great.

Ingredients:

- ½ cup olive oil
- ¼ cup white wine vinegar
- 3 T mayonnaise
- 1 T Worcester sauce
- 1 T lemon juice
- 1 tsp salt
- 1 tsp pepper

Mix all of these ingredients and then coat your pieces of meat with it. The marinade will go very well with a number of different types of meat, including beef, pork, and chicken. Thanks to the oil and mayo, it also adds a few more of those precious calories to the meal for you.

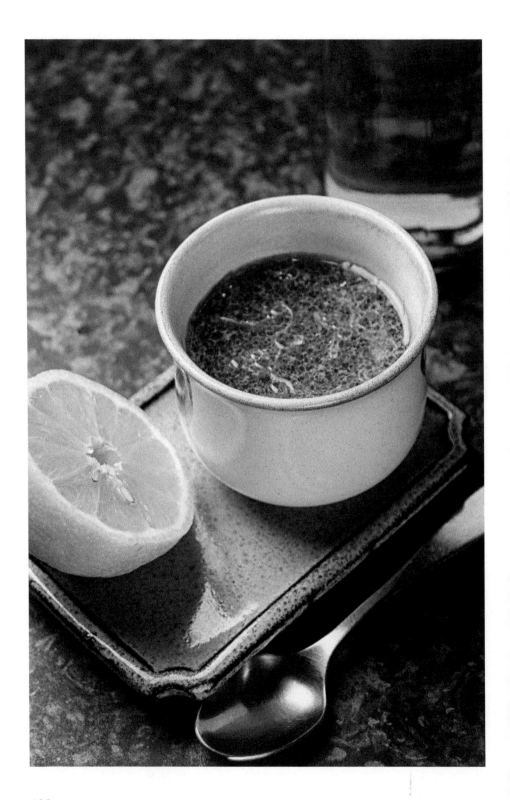

Marinade #2

Here is another marinade recipe that does not include any sugar. It will also work well with a number of different types of meat, and it is just as simple to make as the first.

Ingredients:
- 1 cup vegetable oil or olive oil
- ½ cup soy sauce
- ¼ cup apple cider vinegar
- ¼ cup lemon juice
- 1 T mustard – your choice
- 3 T Worcester sauce

Simply mix up all of these ingredients and then coat your meat with it. Leave it marinating for a minimum of an hour in the refrigerator before cooking.

Both of these marinades are very simple and have only a handful of ingredients. As you progress and learn more about the herbs and spices you can handle, you will then be able to add to the recipes to make them your own and to suit your tastes.

Summary

The drinks you ingest do not have to be boring, and you do not have to give up on all of your favorites. You can have iced coffee without all of the sweet "junk" the chain stores put into it, and you can create an entire book full of your own smoothie recipes since there are so many options out there today! Combine different fruits, peanut butter, and more. By adding just a bit of additional protein powder to your smoothies, you get even more from them, so don't neglect this important tip!

When it comes to marinades, they can be a great way to add both more flavor and a few more calories to your meat. You can put them on chicken, beef, pork, and even fish if you want. You can even turn some of the marinades into a dip for your vegetables, too. Use them whenever you can, and experiment to develop your own unique recipes.

Once again, you should be able to see that just because you are eating differently now, it does not mean you are eating boring in any way, shape, or form! Make your meals exciting, and it really can make getting back into the swing of eating quite a bit easier.

CHAPTER 10

Dealing With Social Gatherings after Gastrectomy

One of the things few people think about and even fewer discuss after a gastrectomy is how they can get back to "normal" when it comes to the social functions in their life. Whether it is simply going back to work and talking with coworkers or going out to lunch, visiting family for holiday meals, or heading over to a friend's house to watch the big game, things will be different.

It is very important to remember that your gastrectomy will likely alter how you approach these gatherings. After all, you will not be celebrating with cake every week when someone at your office has a birthday. You won't be eating cake at family birthday celebrations, either.

This can actually affect quite a few different elements of your life, so it is important to have a plan in place for when these things ultimately come up. Eventually, they will.

How Do You Talk to People... and Should You?

Just as when it comes to the types of foods you can and can't tolerate and the types of foods you like, everyone is different here. After all, eating habits will change quite a bit after the surgery. You will have lost a substantial amount of weight as well, and many may already know that you had cancer.

For those who are going back to work, it may be a good idea to talk to your manager and boss about the situation, so you can let them know why you need to eat throughout the day. Often, they will allow you to have your snacks at your desk or allow you to take breaks so you can eat at the right times.

However, telling people about the gastrectomy and explaining how it affects the diet is easier for some than it is for others.

The Extrovert

Some people feel as though they want to be very open and up-front about the matter. They will tell people, even coworkers they do not really know very well, that they simply can't eat the cake because of their gastrectomy.

They tell their family and friends as well, naturally, and they educate their peers about what it's like to live without a stomach or with just a partial stomach. This does several things for them.

First, it puts them in charge of the information that's out there about their health instead of having others speculate. Second, it ensures that people don't continually try to force them to eat something as they do at many family gatherings and other social outings.

Everyone Else

Of course, some people simply aren't that confident. They don't want others to know about their condition, and they try to keep things as private as they possibly can. In fact, this is how many people feel. This is perfectly natural, and it is perfectly fine.

However, you still must make sure you stick to your dietary plan and don't take those pieces of cake just so you can fit in with the rest of the coworkers, or so you can make your family happy when you visit for the holidays. Your health is still the most important factor, so make sure that you account for that before you account for someone's feelings when you tell them you can't try their cookies.

As awkward as it might be, sometimes just telling people you've had a procedure is the best option.

Dining Out

While you can still dine out, you also need to realize that the way you do it will change, and you have to be far more careful of the things that you order. If you have the time before you go, and ideally you will, make sure you check the restaurant's website to see what they have available—many also include the dish's nutritional information—and compare that to the foods you are currently eating.

Find the offerings that are the most similar and stick to those. You can always choose something small, such as a salad. Just make sure you eat before you get to the restaurant in those cases so you are not losing any calories.

At Home

Your family who lives with you will already know your situation. The family will also know that you are going to be on a different diet plan. It's a good idea to get everyone involved so you can all eat the same sorts of things. Let your family know that just because you won't be eating certain foods, it does not mean that they will not be able to eat them. It's okay if sometimes your meals and snacks differ from theirs.

Getting Additional Help

Sometimes, trying to cope with everything you are going through is difficult, and sometimes you may feel as though you can't—or you do not want to—turn to friends and family for help. Depression and frustration with others can certainly be a contributing factor. It can also be due to you feeling as though you are a "bother" to others.

First, you should never feel as if you are bothering your loved ones. After all, they are your loved ones for a reason! However, if you do feel as though you need to talk to someone who is outside of your usual circle of family and friends, someone who has gone through the same sort of things you have gone through, then you can find online like my website, www.mystomachcancersymptoms.com and offline organizations with which you can connect.

Make an effort to reach out to people in those communities. They are generally very friendly, and they can help you understand how they've been coping after their cancer and gastrectomy. They can let you know how they dealt with social outings and family after it happened, and they can probably even share some of their favorite recipes with you. Sometimes, it is simply nice to have people who really understand who you can speak to.

Summary

How will you handle social situations and dining out after you've had a gastrectomy? Everyone is different, and he or she will want to handle this situation in his or her own way. It will take some practice to get through it.

Sometimes talking with others about the situation is the best course of action, but if that's not always possible or comfortable, at least be sure you are sticking to your new dietary requirements so you can remain healthy. Ultimately, that is what matters.

CHAPTER 11

Develop Your Own Diet Plan and Food Diary

Once you have a basic idea of the types of foods you will be eating, and the quantities you need to eat in order to gain back your weight and to remain healthy, create a diet plan that works for you. Be aware that over time, the diet plan and the foods you eat may evolve.

How to Create a Diet Plan

The first step is to determine what foods you will be eating on your new diet. Earlier in the book, I listed a variety of different food types that you will want to consider. You can choose your own brands, naturally. Just stick to the basics of the list in Chapter 3 in the beginning. Make a list of the foods that you want, as well as the recipes you want to try that incorporate those foods, and then go shopping.

How Many Calories Should Be in the Plan?

When you are building your diet plan, it is a good idea to try to determine the minimum number of calories you need each day in order to regain and then maintain your weight.

Since your weight and your condition are different from everyone else out there, you will need to calculate this on your own. There is no hard and fast rule as to how many calories everyone will need in a day, which makes it impossible to come up with a formula that will work for everyone.

Talk with your physician or dietician for help in this matter to make sure you are eating enough.

The Food Diary

When you write down what you eat, it makes it far easier to gather important data that you can then use to refine and perfect your diet.

What Should You Use?

When it comes to creating your food diary, you can use just about anything you like. If you want to use a notebook and a pen, feel free to do so.

However, it is actually quite a bit faster and easier when you use word processing programs or spreadsheet software, such as Excel. You can even find a free word processor and spreadsheet program through Google or Bing if you don't already have one.

The Type and Amount

Record the type of food that you eat at each meal, along with the amount of food that you eat. Don't forget to include sauces, dips, gravies and drinks.

Record the Calories

Once you know how much food you are eating each day, or at each meal, it becomes easy to determine how many calories you are ingesting in a single setting.

Record the Time of Day

Record the time of day that you are eating, as well as how you feel before and after you have your meals. This is important in determining when your body is best suited to eating. It also helps pinpoint any foods that might be giving your body grief, so you can cut them out of your diet.

Recording Becomes Easier

In the beginning, keeping your food diary is going to feel like a real chore, and it might be one of those chores you forget from time to time. It's important that you keep at it. Eventually, you will remember and it will become like second nature.

Check out the template below for a food diary. You do not have to use this one, but you can develop one that's similar.

Simple Template for a Food Diary

Time of Day	Food	Beverage	How Many Calories?	Feel Before Eating	Feel After Eating

You can also write in longer form in the food diary about how you felt for the day overall. When you go back to your entries later, you will find that it can often clue you into what foods are working well for you, and what foods might be causing problems. Ultimately, this makes it much easier to rework your diet and make it better.

Summary

Keeping a food diary and creating a new diet that will work for your new lifestyle takes some time and some effort, but it is highly worth it. By continually writing in your food diary and by altering your intake when necessary, it is possible to regain the weight you lost and then to maintain a healthy weight, even after going through a gastrectomy.

CHAPTER 12

Tips to Continue Eating Well and Staying Healthy

In this short chapter, I will be going over some very basic and helpful tips I've touched on already in this book. This chapter is merely a refresher and a great way to send you off with the most important information right at the forefront of your mind!

Without further ado, here are ten helpful tips to make sure you eat well and stay healthy after your gastrectomy.

1. Eat foods high in calories and high in nutrition rather than filler foods that make you feel full but that don't have enough calories.
2. Stick to a diet higher in protein.
3. Eat small and frequent meals throughout the day.
4. Carry food with you so you can eat when the time comes, and so you never have to go hungry.
5. Take supplements recommended by your doctor to get additional vitamins.
6. If a food doesn't agree with you or causes dumping syndrome, dump the food!
7. Always look for ways to add calories – butter, gravy, etc.
8. Drink between meals – and try to find drinks that have calories in them.
9. Add protein powder to milk and other drinks.
10. Think of your food as a medicine, especially during those times when you just do not want to eat.

Summary

That's it—ten, quick and to the point tips before you go!

CONCLUSION

You've seen the changes you will be making to your diet, and you've learned more about the potential complications related to eating that could arise after the gastrectomy, not to mention the recipes. So, how do you feel about the changes?

Hopefully, this book has shed some light on the truth behind eating after your surgery, so you have a better idea of what to expect and how to move forward with your life. It does not have to be frightening, nor does it have to overwhelm you.

As I've mentioned before, even though there will be changes, they are changes you can handle, especially with the info gleaned from reading this book.

It's time you put what you learned into action.

ABOUT DR. PETER THATCHER

Peter Thatcher trained as a doctor at Kings College Hospital in London in 1988.

After specialist training, he was appointed as a consultant physician and gastroenterologist at the Royal Cornwall Hospital, Truro, England, in 1995.

Peter has a particular interest in stomach cancer and is the author of the website, www.mystomachcancersymptoms.com, and an information site for sufferers and their families to gain a better understanding of the disease, its course and the treatment options available.

It is not only his wealth of experience in the subject that has made him a leading stomach cancer educator on the Internet, it is also a disease that is close to his heart.

For it was during his clinical training in 1990 that his father, Graham, developed the condition, giving Peter a very personal as well as professional story to tell.

Getting involved, promoting awareness, providing help is so important in the fight against this disease!

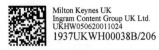